Hair is Hair

How to Nurture, Strengthen and Protect Your Natural Hair Structure

Eugenia Shaw

This book is dedicated to my beautiful daughter Jerene Shaw-Captan. "You've been, and continue to be, my constant motivation, to strive to be a better me, each and every day. You are one of my biggest reasons, I face each and every day with the determination to be the very best version of me. You are my inspiration."

"Happy 20th Birthday!!!"

Contents

Acknowledgements

I would like to say a very big thank you to the wonderful people in my life that encouraged and supported me on this exciting journey. My support team has been absolutely phenomenal. I will treasure you all always.

To my daughter *Jerene*, I say thank you for being my constant inspiration and supporting me through this journey. I also say thank you for walking beside me through it all. I know it wasn't easy. Being a single parent it has meant it's just been the two of us up to this point, and I have treasured every moment.

Philenea Browne, my mother, I thank you for being an amazing role model. Thank you for showing and giving me the strength to be me, in this world.

Omanza Shaw, my dad, thank you for inspiring me with your written word and photographs.

George Smarte, my brother and his husband *Jeffery D Quinn*, thank you for your support and keeping me grounded.

Janvier Richards, thank you for being a wonderful cousin sister. We have definitely shared hair stories. Thank you for your support, not letting distance lessen our bond and being by my side all these years.

Elma Shaw thank you for giving your expert knowledge and guidance to this journey of mine. I greatly appreciate all that you do.

Ann and *Robin Hutchingson* thank you for being such inspirational people, bringing the community together and making me feel utterly welcomed and part of you all. My respect and admiration for you both are beyond words.

My dear friend *Jessica Whitehill* of *Seven Scope Films*, thank you for lending your expert knowledge of writing scripts and of the film industry to this project.

Rowan Hampton thank you for your moral and spiritual support.

Gemma Bull, my editor in chief, thank you for making this book a joy to read.

Philippa Willes thank you for your belief in what the book is offering and spreading the word.

Lynn Abrahams and *Steve Upton* thank you for your support and being such good friends and wonderful neighbours.

Anne Hulbaekdal thank you for your words of encouragement and enthusiasm in the finished product before it was yet started.

Kay Galbraith, artist and illustrator, thank you for your wonderful original watercolour illustrations.

Ann Tanczos of *SciComm Studios* thank you for your wonderful 3D image of keratin on the front cover.

Simone Scott-Sawyer, thank you for doing my very 1st video interview. Your media and interviewing skills made me feel completely at ease.

Nina Cioca, thank you for doing my make-up. You are an amazing make-up artist and it was a joy to teach you your craft.

Jonners Davies thank you being a media wiz and writing up the first public article about me and this book. Your professionalism in getting me relaxed and fired up about my favourite subject 'hair' brought out the best in me.

I thank you all for all that you do, to bring colour, inspiration and richness to my life. Much love to you all, may God richly bless you all always and forever. xxx

Chapter 1

The Journey

Hair is Hair. This is a self help book for anyone who has hair, anyone from any race and with any hair type. You will come to realise by the end of this book, that it doesn't matter what hair type you have or what race you are from, hair needs the same things to perform at its best. Moisture and nutrients.

This book is to help you obtain healthy scalp and hair, and I am very passionate about these two things. With a healthy scalp you will always produce and grow healthy hair; and with healthy hair you will retain length, maintain shine, lusciousness and rock whatever hairstyle you choose. A healthy scalp and healthy hair is the bedrock of good looking hair, period.

The concept of this book will make you question what you think is "normal". My only request is that you lay aside what you have been told, by family, society and culture just for a little bit. After you have heard what I have said, give it some thought, based on the facts, and then make your decision. So many times in life, we take what we have learned and superimpose it on what the facts are. This creates our perception of the situation.

Often times our learned behaviour has been passed down from generation to generation, ingraining it in our "normal" way of life, making our perception fact to us, when in fact, it is just our perception, laid over the true facts. I am coming from a different angle on this, I know. Whilst I absolutely embrace diversity, ethnicity, being Black, being different, I would like to do away with the difference and show you how we are actually not so different from each other after all, and this includes our hair.

Our hair may look different, 'look' being the operative word, but structurally it isn't. If that's the case, then all hair needs the same things to function properly. Let me ask you this; "When a heart surgeon learns how to operate on the heart, does he learn what a Black person's heart looks like and what a Caucasian person's heart looks like, and how to operate on them in their different ways? Or does he just learn how a heart works and learns how to fix it? Do dermatologists learn how the skin and hair function, or do they learn what a Black person's skin and hair does and what an Asian person's skin and hair does?" The purpose of our skin and hair on our body does not change from race to race.

Yes, we may have some biological differences due to external evolutionary factors that have had a part in playing how our genes function, and this is what causes us to look different, however, the actual function of the human body and ALL its parts do not change from race to race. All this perceptive difference is brought on by our location and cultural differences. That is not a bad thing; it is what makes each and every one of us unique in our own special way.

This is what absolutely blows my mind; that I am so unique that there is not another me out there, but yet, I am just the same as the next person cellularly and structurally. Our consciousness and how it's shaped is what makes us so very unique, but this body that carries around our consciousness is the same as everyone else's! So all hair is the same, cellularly and structurally. Hair is hair!

"Surely there is a reason our hair looks different, Eugenia?" I hear you ask. Of course hair looks different from one person to another. The reason for this is genes. The condition your body is in, medically fit or unwell, will also play a big part in how your skin and hair looks, and the different stages in our lives where there are a lot of hormones coursing round the body will have an impact as well. Take pregnancy and puberty for example. Some women find during pregnancy their hair growth rate speeds up, others find their hair falls out and still others like me find their hair stops growing all together, until all the pregnancy hormones have left their bodies.

Genes determine the colour of your hair, the texture of your hair, how curly or straight it is, the thickness of your hair strands, the length of your hair growth cycle, the level of porosity your hair has, the amount of hair you have on your head and lots more. However, genes do not change or determine the type of cells that make up hair and skin. The type of cells that make them up and the way these cells are put together (structure), are the same in every single human being on this planet. Bearing this in mind, this book is all about how anyone from any race and any background can achieve healthy hair, or good hair as it is commonly referred to.

This brings us to the question, "What is good hair?" Amongst the Black population this question comes up at least a few times daily. I have been told, on many occasions by lots of different people, whilst I'm giving advice to them, that their hair cannot achieve whatever I'm advising, and when I ask why not, they say it's because they do not have good hair.

Quite recently, "on my birthday last year in fact," I was told by a lady that my family had good hair and she was envious, that she wished she had hair like ours. My question to her was "Well... what is good hair?" She could not answer me, and so we entered into a discussion about what 'good hair' was and by the end she was a little convinced that there is no such thing as good hair. So I pose that same question to you, "What is good hair? What does good hair look like?"

She was only a little convinced because of culture and years of hand-me-down information on what 'good hair' is supposed to look like, and that mental store of information influenced and continues to influence her perception of what 'good hair' is.

To answer this question correctly we have to reframe the question and ask *"What is our perception of good hair?"* I will ask this question again at the end and see if you have a different answer to what you have now.

For a majority of the world's population, both males and females, the hair on their head is seen as their crowning glory. For Black women all over the world this is especially true. Since our hair is perceived differently by everyone including ourselves, we are sometimes afraid or unsure of our hair. Apart from skin colour, hair is the other thing that sets us apart.

During the slave years, growing one's hair was seen as defiant, and because according to the slave masters our hair looked like animal hair they presumed our hair would have parasites in it, so the slaves were made to cut off their hair. This was not the case, however. It was the very depraved and unsanitary conditions slaves were kept in that made parasitic infections of the hair and body in Black slaves commonplace, and led most slave masters to believe that Black people always had parasites on them and in their hair.

Most people are scared of, fascinated by, and apprehensive of the unknown and unfamiliar. Black hair falls into this category.

This curiosity fuels the big question…. "To touch or not to touch?" a Black person's natural hair. Funnily enough most Black men know not to touch a Black woman's hair… regardless of hairstyle. This is because he has grown up with mother, aunties and or sisters, and has seen these women in his life take their time and spend a LOT of money to get their hair to be just the way they want it to be. They have also heard the stories retold of the bad things that happened to men in these women's lives when they risked or accidentally touched their hair, so… he knows not to touch! However, people will see a Black woman with natural hair and dive right in, dirty hands and all.

I tell you an interesting story that happened to me. I was at a birthday party in London. I had styled my hair into a fro and my curls were popping. My hair looked healthy, shining and my curls were on point! I felt good, and felt I looked beautiful. When I got to the party, I met my friend and she took me round and introduced me to her friends. As we started greeting people, everyone was saying how amazing my hair was looking.

As I greeted this one lady with a casual handshake and a cheek to cheek touch, she suddenly let go of my hand and before I knew what was happening, I felt both her hands in my hair, either side of my face, with a scrunching massaging motion, as she cooed "oh my god I just love your hair". I was absolutely shell-shocked and trapped in between her hands.

There were a lot of things going through my mind at that moment. "My hair is clean! I've just washed my hair, and now you've put your dirty hands straight into my clean hair. I don't know where your hands have been. Where you have been before this party? Have you been to the toilet, shook a lot of people's hands? Handling money, drinks, snacks, eating food? I'm not sure how clean your hands are to be in my hair!!! They are most certainly not clean enough according to my standards, for touching my hair!

Who even give you permission to touch my hair! You didn't ask!!! How very insulting! You are ruining my carefully crafted hairstyle! Now I have to restyle and reshape my hair! Oh good Lord!" This was my mental rant.

Ok, ok, ok, so she's touched your hair with her dirty hands and ruined your hairstyle, do you let it slide or do you say something? All this went through my head in a space of about 5 seconds!

Prior to her touching my hair that night, unsolicited touching of my hair had happened on different occasions and I was debating how to respond to such things were it to happen again. I wanted people to realise that it is not ok to touch anyone's hair, especially a Black person's hair, without their permission! This is because once it is styled, (and a lot of work goes into it), anything that messes with the hair changes the style or ruins it, and this even includes the wind. So deliberately ruining a Black person's hair is not exactly the best way to build up your friendship with them now, is it?

So I decided "enough is enough, I am going to say something". Seeing as I was still trapped between her hands, I leaned back to her ear and said, "You do realise that it is inappropriate to do that, don't you?" And her response was, "Oooo.... but I just love 'your' hair. It feels so fluffy and I just can't help myself, I just want to touch it all the time! It feels so nice!". All this time her hands are still scrunching and massaging my hair all over! To which I respond, "But that still doesn't make it ok to do so, it's still inappropriate." It was then that she finally pulled her hands from my hair, almost reluctantly, and "kind of confusedly" said; "Oh... I'm sorry I didn't realise." She then proceeded to tell me how she's got nephews and nieces with 'our' hair type and she just loves touching it. She apologised again and I moved on.

I put my bag and coat down and raced to the bathroom to make my hair decent once again. That incident put a damper on my night, as I felt mauled and dirty, as if I was some showpiece that people could touch because they wanted to. I decided then, that I would post something on my Facebook page to say it wasn't ok to touch people's hair without their permission. I also determined that I was going to wash my hair that night, to get all the dirt from her hands out of my hair, no matter what time it was when I arrived home after the party. When that was all done, I was crawling into bed around 4:30am, after arriving home at 2am. I'm glad I decided to wash my hair, as I found some brown congealed muck embedded in 3 different parts of my hair! The most disgusting my hair has ever felt. I felt angry... why should I have to be hassled into washing my hair because of someone's ignorance?

After my Facebook post, it then became the in-house joke for people to ask me, whenever they saw me, "Can I touch your hair?", which is a kind of ignorant statement in itself, as they are completely missing the point, which is "Ask permission if you want to touch," but it however, opened a dialogue platform for people to engage with the issue and talk about it. From then on people stopped touching my hair! Result achieved... yes!

The problem most Black people face with regards to touching their hair is this: nobody asks! Everyone presumes it's ok to go ahead and touch their hair because they want to touch it and they don't see why the Black person should mind. Black people do mind, because when you touch their hair without permission you are instantly disrespecting them, because you are saying, "I don't care about how you feel or what your decision is! I am satisfying my curiosity, and that's all that matters in this instance."

However, what you will find is most Black people don't mind you touching their hair if you ask their permission. Black people are curious too about Caucasian hair you know. But they don't randomly touch a Caucasian's or Asian's hair, they ask or admire from afar. So if you are curious about a Black person's hair and would like to touch (not stroke... like a zoo animal), here's what you could say... "I'm curious about the difference between your hair and mine, the way your hair is fascinates me. Would you be terribly offended if I asked you to please touch your hair?" What you will find with an approach like that, is, most Black people will let you touch. There will be some who will say no, and that is perfectly alright. Most importantly though, you need to respect that decision and accept it. Best not to launch into a debate about how you don't understand why they won't let you touch their hair. That decision is theirs, and only theirs to make, and honestly, it will have nothing to do with you. *It is all about how the person feels about letting people touch their hair.*

Do not also forget that some people may have severe allergies; you may have an anaphylactic-shock causing allergen on your hands, and by touching their hair may transfer it to them, causing a mild or severe reaction, when their hair touches their skin, which is a guarantee, as scalp is skin. They may not have allergies but they could transfer what you have transferred to them to someone else who has an allergy.

I was talking to a Caucasian friend and client of mine, about this same scenario and the conversation was very interesting. She made an interesting point which I absolutely love. Her point was "How is it that most races inherently know not to go up to another person (random or not) and start stroking or touching their hair, yet other races are still having this conversation?" What is your answer to this question? We all know what to do yet somehow we are still having this discussion. I will leave you with that question and we will leave the rest of that discussion to another book perhaps.

So, the long and short of it all is, ask, and then respect and accept their answer.

However, please, please, please do not walk up to some random stranger in the street or at a party and say this or you might get knocked out! Make sure it's someone you know, a friend or friend of a friend.

I have had a few hair experiences over the years. I do look back on them now with a fondness, if you can call it that, however they were all learning experiences and what catapulted me onto this journey.

Growing up I had a very sensitive scalp, I still do have a sensitive scalp, "it was" prone to bruising, swelling and bleeding, and any number of these things will leave me with a migraine (that would have me crying as a kid) for 24hrs plus. When it wasn't my mom doing my hair, I was always that child that cried when my hair was being done and was always unhappy with the final result. Mostly because detangling was inappropriately done and so by the time we came to plaiting, my scalp was so swollen that any plaits, let alone really tight ones, brought on my migraines. But being in Africa..., Liberia, West Africa to be precise, it was all pegged down to me being a difficult child that didn't like to have her hair done. Worst of all, I had thick long hair, so, very difficult to manage. More often than not, I would be in so much pain and be so miserable that my mom would come from work and have to redo my hair. Only my mom knew how to do my hair so that it didn't irritate my scalp. Because I would always get my mom to redo my hair after it was done by someone else, I was pegged as a spoilt brat. I don't think my mom realised the severity of my scalp condition, she just knew her days and nights would be absolute misery if she didn't redo my hair, so she did. Even I didn't know the full extent of my scalp condition until I started doing my own hair and researching why I had the problems I had with my scalp.

I, like everyone else at the time, accepted that I was the problem, I had difficult hair, and I was the fussy one, only wanting my mom to do my hair. I used to remember thinking "There has to be a better way than this!" However, I used to just give in, because everyone around me said or implied that that was normal. I remember this one time my mom's cousin or friend (I can't exactly remember which) came round to visit for a few days. It was busy at the hospital where my mom worked, and she had washed my hair with the intention to plait but had been called into work that day. It was the visitor's last day with us and as my mom had been called in she offered to plait my hair for my mom. (People were always offering to plait my hair. It almost seemed that the more I didn't want anyone other than my mom to plait my hair, the more offers she got.)

It was Sunday and my mom wanted my hair to be ready for school on Monday, so she agreed, knowing she wouldn't have time to plait it when she came back from work. Off my mom went off to work and the stool was pulled out for me to sit on. I do remember asking this lady to not plait my hair tight, please. And her response was, "It won't be neat for school then." And I said "But it hurts." She just laughed and said "Oh you'll be fine." My mom had already asked her to do really big plaits and she had agreed to do only five big cornrows on my head. So down I sat and the plaiting began. Thirty to forty five minutes later the plaiting was done, I said thank you and ran off behind the house to cry.

When she was ready to leave she asked for me, and the housekeeper came and got me. I was in my bedroom, eyes all puffy. She asked what was wrong and the housekeeper said that I always did this when someone else other than my mom plaited my hair, so it was nothing to worry about. She said her goodbyes and left. The minute she left I went back into my bedroom with the intention of undoing all of my hair.

I tell you, to this day my hair has never ever been plaited so tight as it was then, [*not even when I had my first weave as an adult and that was tight then!*] This lady had plaited my hair so tight that it felt like my skin was being lifted off my scalp. It was tightest at the beginning and at the end. So my face felt lifted and pulled so tight I couldn't close my eyes properly. My hair at the nape of my neck was also so tight I couldn't actually turn my head from side to side.

All I wanted to do was relieve this pressure that was building. I got into my bedroom, shut the door behind me and quickly found my comb. I started to undo the hair, but this lady had plaited my hair so tight I couldn't even get the comb through the ridge gaps in the plait. Well..., there should have been ridge gaps, but there were none! I was frustrated and in pain and by now had had enough. I turned, went to get my mom's sewing scissors..., came back and sat in front of the mirror in my bedroom and proceeded to cut off my hair! I just wanted relief in the front of my hair and the back, so I cut the beginning and the end of each plait, away from my scalp. I tried not to cut too close to the scalp because I knew I was doing irreparable damage and I would be in big trouble when my mom got home that evening, so I wanted to minimise the damage. I knew all of this and I still went ahead and cut my hair...., that's how much pain I was in. I only cut up to where and when the relief began, my whole head hurt but I only cut until the worst part had subsided at the front and back. The next morning I was too afraid to get up and get ready for school, so I waited for my mom to come and wake me. I was too afraid to see the look on her face when she saw and realised what I had done. Mostly because I was afraid of what punishment I would get, but also, I didn't want to see my mom upset!

When she saw my hair she was horrified. I explained what had happened and she said not to worry and that she would undo the hair to see what real damage was done. My hair being so tight, coupled with the swelling of my scalp made a 10-minute job take an hour. It looked like someone had used my head as a punching bag, she had to touch it very softly. From that day on, my mom never let anyone do my hair again.

That was the day the urgency for learning how to do my own hair was born. The question "Why do we do hair this way.

Why is this normal, when it is so obviously not right?" surfaced and stayed with me.

When I had my weave done for the first time as an adult, it was so tight I had a migraine that lasted a week. It started me thinking "I need to learn how to do hair, because I don't accept that this is the right way. Since everyone around me accepts it as it is, if I don't learn it to change it, change will never come." However, my desire to become a vet outweighed any desires of becoming a hairdresser. By this time I was already doing hair for friends and family, perfecting my craft of being able to plait any hair, from any race, with the neatness and tightness that it needs to stay neat and last for a long period of time, without the plait being tight on the scalp.

I had made the discovery that hair can be plaited, neat and tidy and last a long time without trying to cause any migraines or any scalp issues. Yes! Result! I was happy to do this as a hobby and pursue my career as a vet. When I arrived in the UK, due to financial constraints my career as a vet was put on hold. I carried on doing beauty treatments and hairdressing for friends as a hobby and did different sales and admin jobs. It was when my daughter joined me in the UK that I realised that I could not carry on in the 40hr per week admin job I was doing at the time with a four year old at home.

This is when I trained as a beauty therapist and my hobby became my career.   Every little baby step and giant leap has led me to where I am today and will continue to lead me to where I need to be in this industry to offer the maximum help to others. All of these experiences have fueled my desire to help people have healthy scalp and hair.

Chapter 2

Anatomy and Physiology of Hair and Scalp

- ➢ Structure of the Hair
- ➢ Hair Growth Cycle
- ➢ Hair Porosity
- ➢ Structure of the Skin

There are many books dedicated to the anatomy and physiology of hair and skin but in order to continue, here is a bit of background to give you a better understanding of how and why your hair behaves the way it does. More importantly to help you answer that nagging question "What is our *perception* of good hair?" The key is in the word perception! Whatever is happening around us, what we are told about our hair, how our hair is treated, all contribute to how we perceive where we sit on the good hair bad hair scale. And the answer to that question is "It is all perception. There is no such thing as good hair or bad hair; there is just healthy hair or unhealthy hair! Nothing more, nothing less." Continue reading and you will understand why.

Hair is Hair

Hair is hair... right? What does that mean? Well... it means that when you look at the structure and cell composition of the hair and scalp, from any race, under the microscope it looks the same! It is made up of the same cells, the cells have the same structure and the way they bond and sit together is exactly the same! Woah....! Wow...! This just blows my mind. Did you know that? The hair and scalp biologically and structurally looks exactly the same and behaves in exactly the same way across races. So, Black, Asian, Caucasian, Eskimo, we ALL have the SAME hair! However, it looks different due to some minor differences of some of the structures within the scalps of different races brought about by the evolutionary ecological differences in our climates of where we are from. Keep reading and you'll find out how.

I came to this realisation early in my teaching career, after only teaching for a few months. However, I had been working in the Beauty Industry for over 10 years by then and had been doing hair in some way shape or form since my teenage years. Growing up and as an adult it is drummed into you that Black hair is different, Asian hair is different and Caucasian hair is different. Whilst all the time, since man began... it has never been different! It just looks different. How many times have you been given the same thing or tried something over and over again, told it was different every time because it looked different, but then further down the line you realise it's the same thing, just repackaged or the ingredients rearranged in a different order, but same ingredients nonetheless. It is then that you realise you've been duped. This is the same for the age old myth about the different races hairs.

I was going through a consultation with a new private client of mine for hair health, and the age old question of why some races' hair is 'better' than others came up. As I started to answer her, I remembered my lesson I had taught a few days earlier, on hair and skin, and as I tried to explain to her, the realisation came to me that hair is hair! Structurally, how it's formed, how it looks under the microscope and what it requires is no different from race to race. It just requires those things in different orders and different consistencies, but requires the same things nonetheless.

The hair on our head is of the group of hair termed terminal hairs. These are deep rooted hairs that have high pigmentation and texture (compared to the other 2 types of hair, vellus and lanugo). Vellus hair is the soft downy hair we have on some parts of our bodies, like the sides of the face. Lanugo hair is the hair that is on a foetus' body whilst in the womb. This hair is normally all shed by the time the baby is born, however, some babies are born with their lanugo hair and this soon sheds within the first two months.

Hair grows out of structures called follicles, and it is within the hair follicles that the hair bulb, which is part of the hair root, is connected to the blood supply that transports nutrients and hormones necessary for hair growth. The bulb is also connected to the nerve supply, which is why we feel it if our hair is tugged. The hair root is within the hair follicle, and the hair follicle is within the skin. It is the shape of the follicle that determines the shape of the hair and its texture.

There are basically two shapes, round and oval. A round hair follicle will produce straight hair which is structurally round, and an oval follicle will produce curly hair, the flatter the circumference of the follicle, the curlier the hair. I have included four diagrams here for you to see the difference between a round follicle, an oval follicle, a flat oval and a flatter oval follicle.

Shape of the hair, the follicle and angle of the follicle

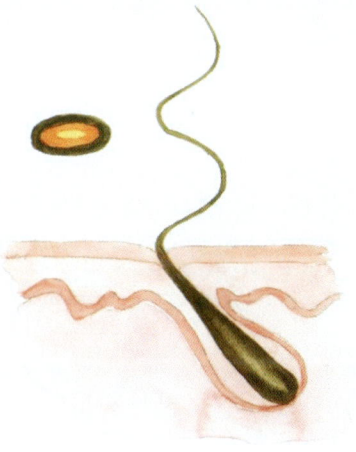

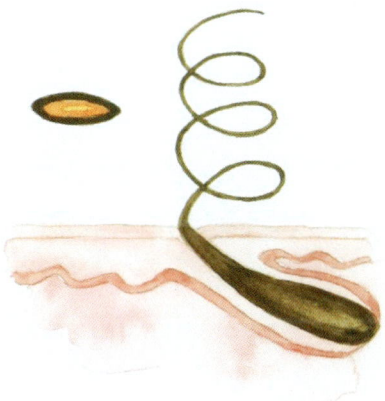

Slightly flat oval shaped & slightly angled follicle produces wavy hair

Flat oval shaped & a much angled follicle produces kinky curly hair

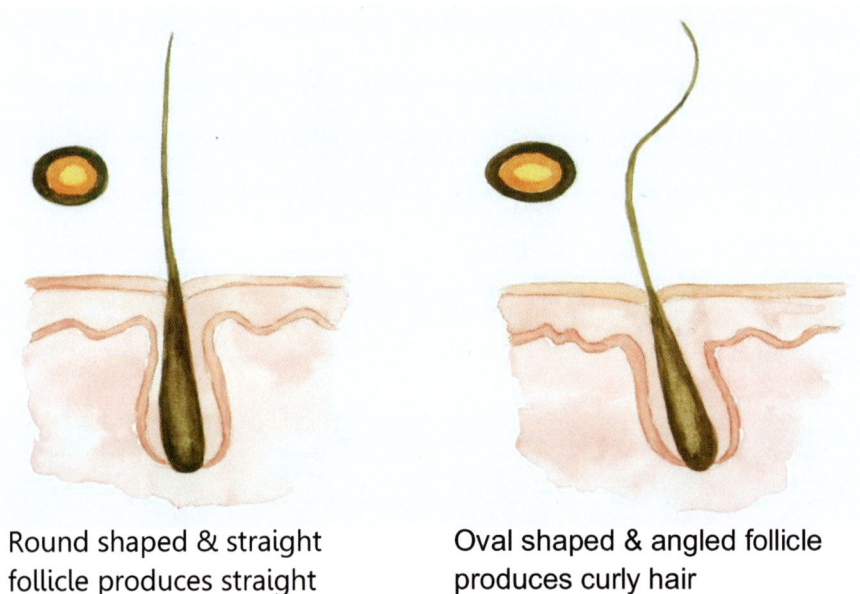

Round shaped & straight
follicle produces straight
hair

Oval shaped & angled follicle
produces curly hair

The shape of the hair follicle and the angle of the hair follicle play an important role in hair type and texture.

A flatter oval shaped hair follicle and angled hair follicle is indicative of Black hair. This structure of hair is the weakest of the four different hair types, due to its flat nature, which makes it curl tightly upon and around itself. These curls do not allow the sebum that is naturally produced by the sebaceous glands in the hair follicles to travel along the hair shaft. There are two reasons for this, #1 because the oil is not travelling at a speed it cannot go around and over the curl, and #2 because of the curls, the hair does not hang down. Curlier hair is drier because the lack of sebum along the hair shaft means no moisturisation to seal the cuticles, causing continuous moisture loss in varying degrees based on the condition of the hair. This makes it more prone to being damaged. This hair type will have an oilier scalp due to the sebum not travelling too far down the hair shaft. This hair type needs a lot of external nourishment to keep length and stay healthy. Does that make this hair type weaker? No not necessarily so, as healthy hair from any race will have the same strength if tested like for like. It is just more susceptible to being damaged.

The oval shaped hair is indicative of Mongolian (wavy to curly Caucasian, Asian and Eskimo) hair. This type of hair has the same issues as the flatter oval shaped hair but not to the same degree. The hair will suffer dryness but not as significant as the above hair type. They will also have oilier scalp due to the sebum not travelling too far down the hair shaft. This hair type needs external nourishment to keep length and stay healthy.

The round shaped hair is indicative of straight Asian, Caucasian and Eskimo hair. The sebum that is produced by this hair type can reach from root to tip with ease. People with this hair type normally say they have a tendency to have greasy hair, and depending on their sebum production it can take anything from 2 to 7 days for their hair to feel greasy in varying degrees. This hair needs maintenance and nourishment to keep hair length and be healthy.

Another contributing factor to the way the hair will curl is the way the follicle burrows into the scalp. Straight hair follicles burrow vertically down into the skin from the skin's surface. The oval shaped follicles burrow into the skin at an angle. The hair curves as it grows out of this angled follicle and that is what causes it to curl.   Along with the follicle shape and the angle of the follicle, another factor which determines how curly hair is, is the sulfur bonds found between the molecules in cells in the hair. These are called disulfide bonds. Curly hair is formed because of the angle and shape of the follicle, allowing different parts of the hair shaft to come closer together, making these disulfide bonds easier to form. Curly hair has more disulfide bonds.

Products (chemicals) that perm hair to either straighten or curl it take advantage of these bonds by either relaxing or breaking them down, or encouraging the disulfide bonds to form. To go from straight to curly you need a chemical to allow the bonds to form, and to go from curly to straight you need a chemical that relaxes or breaks up these bonds.

Structure of the hair

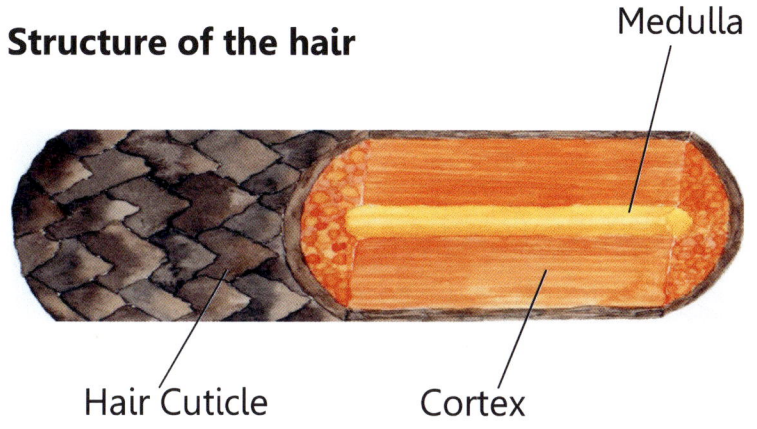

Medulla

Hair Cuticle   Cortex

The hair on our head is there to protect our head, by cushioning it against knocks and blows, and to provide insulation against the cold by working with the blood supply to maintain body temperature. The hair is made up of tough keratinized (hardened) cells and it is an appendage of the skin. There are no nerve endings in the hair shaft, which is why when we cut our hair we do not feel pain.

Hair is made up of three parts; it has a core called the medulla, a thick middle bit called the cortex and an outer sheath called the cuticle. The cuticle is the bit we see. The 3 layers functioning together give hair its strength and flexibility.

The core medulla is the innermost part of the hair and is only present in thick and or coarse hair. The thick cortex middle gives the hair its strength, and this is where pigmentation (hair colour) is held. As we age we lose this colour within the cortex and the hair appears colourless. The colourless hair sitting amongst the coloured hair appears grey. The cuticle is the outermost layer and is comprised of hard scale-like cells that overlap each other. This outer layer works to prevent damage to the inner layers and control the amount water content in the hair shaft.

When we want to effect change, such as colour or deep conditioning, to our hair shaft, we need to do this to the thick middle bit, the cortex. To get at the middle bit, the chemicals or products we apply to our hair softens and raises the cuticles, allowing the chemicals or products to penetrate into the cortex to effect change. This is what happens when we colour, perm, chemically straighten, Brazilian blow dry, condition, deep condition, or give ayurvedic or other treatments to our hair. The conditioning treatments strengthen and nourish the hair shaft, creating healthy hair.

When it comes to colouring our hair, there is no such thing as colour for Afro hair, colour for Mongolian hair, or colour for Caucasian hair. I can see the shocked looks on your faces, but let me explain.

First things first, what we do have to remember is Hair is Hair! As hair is hair and biologically behaves in the same way, any chemicals or products will affect it the same way. When it comes to colouring, people in different parts of the world have used, for centuries, plants, clays and synthetic materials to colour their hair. Some of these products are native to a particular region of the world. Regardless of whether these products have spread over the world or not, they all colour hair the same way. An activator is mixed with colour pigmentation to activate the microscopic colour molecules to cause them to swell. This mixture is placed on the hair, the activator softens and raises the cuticles, and the tiny colour molecules pass through the cuticles and enter into the cortex, where they continue to swell until they are too large to pass out through the cuticles, embedding the colour in the cortex and changing the colour of your hair.

The intensity of colour is based on how many pigment molecules can enter the hair shaft. The more pigment molecules in the cortex, the more intense the colour, the less pigment molecules the duller the colour. The activator will only work for a period of time. That length of time determines when the pigment molecules reach their full swollen size. This time is what is termed 'colour development time'. The shorter the activation period and the larger the pigmentation molecule size, the less permanent the colour. The longer the activation period and the smaller the pigmentation molecules, the more permanent the colour. The size of the pigmentation molecules determines how quickly they can pass through the cuticles into the cortex. Hair loses colour over time because some of the pigmentation molecules shrink back to their original size and pass out the cuticle when we wash our hair. Now, when we understand that hair is hair, and this process is identical for any and every hair texture and type, we understand that there is no such thing as colour just for Afro hair, just for Caucasian hair or just for Mongolian hair. There is just colour, colour that colours hair, and because hair is hair, any colour is for everyone!

Colour pigmentation is made up of different ingredients, and we just have to watch out for the colour intensity we want in our natural hair colour when we colour. For example, colours that are traditionally and culturally produced for Black hair types will have a higher pigmentation ratio due to the fact that most of that hair's type natural colour is jet black, black or off black, so a lighter haired person will have to leave the colour on for a very short period of time to achieve the same results.

Once I was advising a friend on what colour to buy for her hair. When I mentioned the brand for her to get, her response was "Isn't that colour for Caucasian hair?" I tried to explain that she could use it too but I'm not sure I was clear enough. I did however, convince her to buy it, based on the recommendation that I had used that colour brand before.

It got me thinking and I realised I had faced this same question time and time again, from all different sides of the coin. "Isn't that colour just for Black people's hair?" "Isn't that colour just for Asian hair?" "Isn't that colour just for Caucasian hair?" No, no, no, colour is colour and hair is hair. It just depends on what colour you want your hair to be and how permanent or intense you want it to be.

As chemicals damage the bonds between the cells in the hair, over time, with inappropriate use and improper care, we can cause irreparable damage to our hair. Also, the use of excessive heat, improper use of tools and excessive manipulation can cause damage to the hair, weakening the integrity of the hair, making it more prone to breakage and split ends, creating dry brittle hair and causing lack of length retention.

However, please be aware that for all hair types, if you process with heat and or chemicals and don't nourish and treat, over time this becomes over processing and excessive. Without a proper nourishing plan for hair, any hair, it will deteriorate and may lead to irreparable damage.

So, all hair types are prone to damage, some more so than others, it just depends on how we treat and care for our hair.

Hair Growth Cycle

All the hairs all over our body grows in cycles that repeat themselves over and over again. With age these cycles slow down and the time interval becomes longer. These cycles are all at different time frames depending on where the hair is on your body. For the purposes of this book we will be focusing on the terminal hair on the head. Every hair on our head is in a different growth stage at any given moment. About 85% of our scalp hair is in the active growing stage, the other 15% is split between the catagen and telogen stages at any time. This hair growth cycle accounts for why hair sheds!

Hair grows in three different stages: anagen, catagen and telogen stages. There is a fourth stage which is the exogen or evacuation stage, and this is when the hair falls or is pulled out.

Anagen: this is the active growing stage, when the hair bulb of the hair is connected to the blood supply to receive its nutrients to help it grow. The blood supply to the hair bulb is called the dermal papilla and sits in the cavity of the hair bulb. When the new hair bulb starts to form around the blood supply before it is seen on the surface of the skin, after the old hair has fallen out or been pulled out, this is called the early anagen stage.

The anagen stage for the hair on our head can last anything from 2 to 7 years, therefore, no single hair strand grows continuously, and this stage determines the ultimate length of hair that can be achieved by any individual.

This is the stage at which we can affect any change, for longer, healthier hair if we so tried, with treatments and nourishment that increases the blood supply to the hair follicle. By providing vital oxygen and nutrients to the growing hair, we may be able to impact the speed of growth to increase length of hair, but not the length of the anagen stage. The amount of hair growth that takes place in the anagen stage is dependent upon genes, however the flattest oval shaped hair is the slowest growing out of the 4 shapes and the round shaped hair is the fastest growing. People of mixed heritage have a blended growth length. If the ends of the hair are also simultaneously nourished to make sure they are not breaking off, we will see an increase in length. The combination of scalp stimulation, nourishment and moisturisation, and nourishment and strengthening of hair shaft, is what will produce healthy long hair.

Catagen: this is the changing stage of the hair, where it begins to separate from the blood supply and the hair follicle prepares to rest.

Telogen: this is the resting stage, where the hair has detached from the blood supply and the base of the follicle degenerates and enters into the resting stage. This stage can last 3 to 4 months. It is at this stage at that hair is shed! (The shedding of the hair is the exogen stage.) However, many follicles do not go into the resting stage but immediately start to produce a new hair, and it is the new hair that pushes out the old hair.

Exogen: this is the stage when the hair is either pushed out by the new hair, brushed or combed out, or falls out naturally or is pulled out after going through the telogen stage.

I would like to touch on shedding for a bit. The hair on your head is in all different stages of growth at any given moment, and we shed hair every day. Now, the amount of hair you shed is dependent on your hair growth cycle (what percentage of your hair is in the telogen stage), and your hair care routine. It is unique to you and you alone!

However when you consider hairstyles that hold hair in any given position for any number of days, you have to be aware that when you do eventually undo that hairstyle, the hair that will be shed or come out is the normal daily shed amount multiplied by the number of days that the hair has been plaited or held in place for. If you have had your hair plaited for 3 days then undo it, there will be three days of shed hair that will come out. The same is true if you've had it plaited for 7 days, 2 months or 4 months.

However, the longer you keep your hairstyle in, the more prone the shed hair is to wrapping around growing hair and matting, creating lots of tangles... yikes. This is especially relevant for anyone who wears braided hairstyles, or anyone wanting to try them out for the first time. The shock is always at the point of undoing the hairstyle, after the first time you had it done. Over time you get adjusted to what is happening and understand it.

I have had many clients call me up in a panic saying, "I'm losing my hair! Is this a normal amount of hair that should be coming out?" Once the above has been explained they are relieved. Or they call me up and say, "Thank God you told me about this shedding thing, because I feel like I'm losing my hair."   As long as there is no underlying condition, it will be a normal shed.

A common misconception is that hair can heal. Only living tissue or cells can heal, and since hair is made up of dead epithelial cells, it stands to reason then, that hair cannot heal itself. However, nourishing treatments can prep and 'bandage' it up until the new hair grows through. If hair is damaged, the damage <u>cannot</u> be undone, but it can be looked after in such a way as to prevent further damage and to manage the current damage. That damage <u>will only</u> go away when that hair falls out and the new hair grows through from the hair follicle. Until then, it is damage-control, literally. To effect any changes to our hair, we need to care, stimulate and nourish our scalp, and implement damage-control and or maintenance measures to our hair shaft. This is how we maintain length and promote new growth.

Sometimes I get people who say to me "Eugenia this is all fair and good but I can never get my hair to grow past a certain length. My hair just stops growing when it gets to this length." This phenomenon is true for all races. Now, as I have mentioned previously, your hair never just stops growing, it goes through a cycle. "So why does it not grow past a certain length?" I hear you ask. This is solely due to the fact that your hair is breaking off at the tip when it gets to that length. Your hair is continuing to grow from your scalp but due to your hair care regime and practices, your hair shaft is breaking off from the tip, making it appear as if it's not growing. Every time it grows from the scalp the same amount of growth breaks off at the tip, thus creating a stagnant length. To change that, you need to reassess your practices for caring for your hair shaft, to strengthen it and keep those cells from breaking off. The products and hairstyles chapter should help you with this.

The above break down, of hair and its functions are exactly the same for all races! Let that sink in for a moment. Yes you read right... There are no biological or anatomical differences in the hair of different races. They are ALL the same. Hair is hair!

Hair porosity and how that affects the way our hair behaves

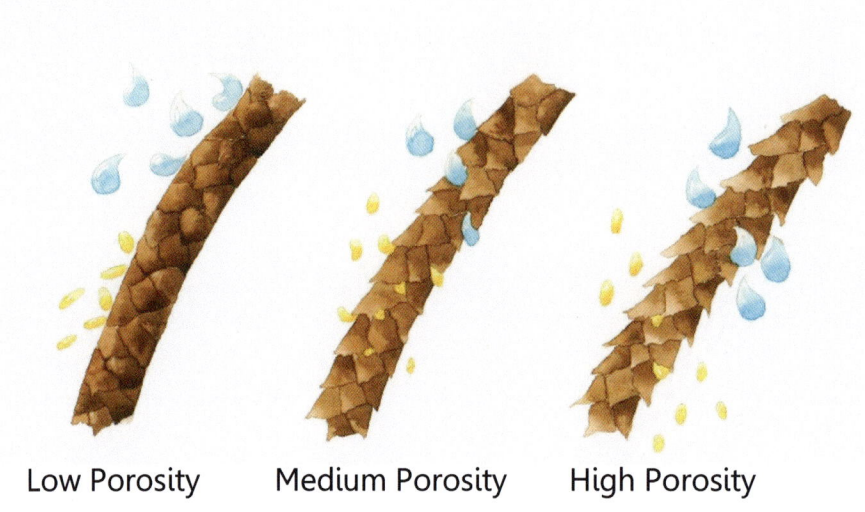

Low Porosity   Medium Porosity   High Porosity

What is hair porosity and what does this mean for your hair?

Porosity of hair simply means, your hair's ability to absorb and retain moisture. Moisture is essential for growth, flexibility and suppleness. Porosity is genetic, however it can be affected by external factors, good and bad, factors such as a change in climate, exposure to heat treatments and or chemical processing. Being aware of your hair's porosity will help you in choosing the right products, treatments and chemical processing for your hair.

Hair cuticles that are tightly closed allow little to no moisture to enter into the hair shaft. This hair has very low porosity. It is characterised by coarseness, and prone to dryness, easily breaks, may have a shiny appearance.

Hair cuticles that are lying flat but not tightly closed allows for some moisture to enter the hair shaft. This hair has normal porosity, allowing just the right amount of water it needs in and retaining that moisture. We want to strive for our hair to be in this category. It is characterised by a shiny appearance, soft and supple, and not dry.

Hair cuticles that are raised allow too much moisture into the hair shaft, however, it loses that moisture just as quickly, because of the raised cuticles moisture and products are able to enter quickly but are also evaporated just as quickly. It is characterised by dull lacklustre hair, it is dry, breaks off and sheds easily. This is indicative of over processed damaged hair.

Porosity does not determine length of hair but can affect how long hair is able to grow.

How to test and find out the porosity of your hair?

Float test: take a couple of strands of hair from your comb or brush, place in a bowl of room temperature/ mildly lukewarm water. Leave for about two to four minutes. If your hair sinks it has high porosity, if it floats it has low porosity. If it half sinks and floats, you have normal porosity.

Slip and Slide test: take a strand of your hair, still attached to your head or from your comb or brush (you would need to work out which end is the root and which end is the tip if you take from the comb or brush). Pinch the hair strand between thumb and forefinger and slide your fingers from tip to root. If it feels bumpy or catchy, you have normal to high porosity hair. The more bumpy the hair the higher the porosity. if it slides smoothly, you have medium to low porosity hair.

As you have come to realise, hair does look different, but that's because it grows slightly differently. However, it is made up of the same things and requires the same things, so there is no such thing as good hair or bad hair, <u>there is just healthy hair that looks good and unhealthy hair that looks bad</u>. Find out what your scalp and hair needs to be healthy and then do it as often as required!

Most of what we feel about or perceive of our hair and other people's hair is based on learned behaviour; from the media and the people around us, our culture, upbringing and all the ancestral knowledge passed down. A good perception of and healthy practices is all it takes to have 'good hair'. The *key,* being healthy practices, which without these you will not have good looking hair. Chapters 3, 4 and 5 teach you how to instil healthy practices in your hair care regime to help you have 'good hair'.

When someone asks you what is good hair, especially if that someone is your child or someone that looks up to you,

you will now be able to give an uplifting, nurturing answer that helps them be proud of what their hair looks and feels like, and help them manage it too.

See.... our prejudices, racial, religious etc..., have kept us from seeing what is actually there, in fact what has been there since the beginning of man; hair is hair, regardless of race, colour or origin.

Structure of the skin

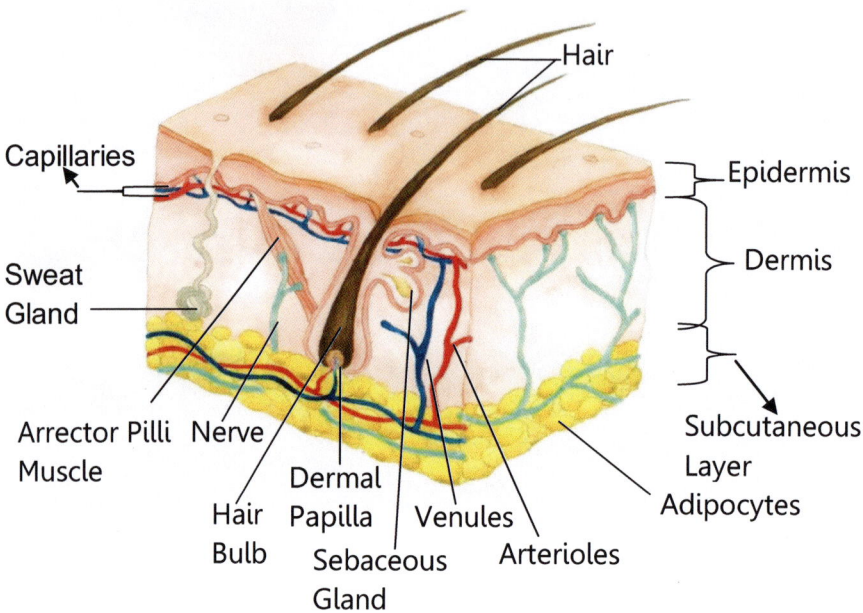

Capillaries

Hair

Epidermis

Dermis

Sweat Gland

Arrector Pilli Muscle

Nerve

Hair Bulb

Dermal Papilla

Sebaceous Gland

Venules

Arterioles

Subcutaneous Layer

Adipocytes

We include and talk about skin here; because the hair on our head grows out of the portion of our skin we call the scalp. The same care and diligence spent on our skin elsewhere on our body, needs to be implemented for our scalp, which is skin.

Our skin is the largest organ in our body and that is in both surface area and weight. It is made up of three layers that work together and function as one organ.

The outermost layer, the epidermis is made up of five sub-layers. It is the very top sub-layer of this layer that we can see and touch, the stratum corneum or horny layer as its commonly know.

The middle layer is the dermis, often referred to as the true skin. This is made up of two sub-layers. This layer contains the blood supply, nerve endings and fibrous supportive and connective tissues.

The bottom layer is the subcutaneous layer. This is a layer of fat cells whose primary function is to protect the underlying tissues and organs, act as a food store and regulate body temperature. All three layers together make up the skin. The skin's primary functions are protection, absorption, excretion, secretion and heat regulation.

The skin produces sebum, which mixes with our sweat and forms the acid mantle, which is the skin's chemical barrier, with a slightly acidic pH around the mark of 5.5. If it is a few points below or above this number then we have scalp problems. One of the many reasons people have scalp problems, is due to the acid mantle on the scalp being compromised. This disturbance can be caused by products and or chemicals, or the introduction of fungi, viruses, and or bacteria.

Diseases, Disorders and Infections that can affect the scalp are many, but to name a few, excessive dandruff, folliculitis (infection of the hair follicles that can be caused by fungus, bacteria and viruses with symptoms such as swelling, pus in the hair follicle, pain and itching); lice (pediculosis capitis), a parasitic infection of the hair and scalp; psoriasis and eczema of the scalp; and fungal infections of the scalp which are highly infectious and can spread to the whole family if care is not taken. For any disease, disorders and infection, medical intervention is needed, even if it is holistic in nature. Some form of treatment of the problem needs to take place to get rid of the problem.

The symptoms of scalp problems include dull looking hair, dry and brittle, rough or coarse, excessive itching, redness, soreness, burning sensation, bad or 'funny' smell, too much dead skin, excessive shedding, stagnant growth, bald patches or loss of hair. If your scalp is manifesting any such symptoms, you have a problem. Please go and see a doctor and let them run some tests to find out what is wrong and start treating it. This is the only way these symptoms will stop and your hair can then start recovering, then you can move into hair growth and healthy looking hair.

Black hair types are prone to fungal, bacterial and viral infections. This is because most of the sebum produced sits on the 10% of hair closest to scalp. The hair is so curly it blocks out light, traps sweat and heat, creating a dark moist greasy area. These combinations of conditions are perfect breeding ground for bacteria, fungi and viruses. For Black hair, wigs and weaves exacerbate the problem. We don't have to look far for these microorganisms, as everyone has them living naturally on the skin, in a harmony of good and bad of each, creating perfect equilibrium, thus insuring we have healthy skin and hair. The above conditions make the bad bacteria, fungi and viruses multiply and overwhelm the good microorganisms creating an imbalance, and in the process destroying the acid mantle. It is this imbalance that produces the problems.

Fungal infections are the most common and most detrimental to Black hair, however, most Black people don't notice until hair loss is significant, or the other symptoms are amplified. Sometimes there will be an initial infection that will cause major problems immediately, but more often than not, the problem starts off small, one tiny little spot on your scalp and before long it becomes normal for your hair and scalp to look and feel that way. It slowly spreads, and can be months or even years before the infection is noticed as a problem. By this point in time, the person thinks the condition is 'normal', as their hair has always been that way for as long as they can remember. This can start at a very young age or later on in life.

When these problems already exist, caring for the client's hair as a hairdresser or caring for your own hair with just hair products will be an uphill battle as you will be treating a symptom not the cause. What you have to remember is, the longer these problems exist the more deep rooted (pardon the pun) it becomes, and the longer it will take to get rid of the problem. For any problem to get better it will take twice as long as you have had the problem, so if you have had a fungal infection for about two weeks it will take about four to five weeks once treatment has commenced for it to get better, if you've had it for five years, it'll take 5 to 10 years for the problem to be completely gone. If the infection has been there for years, it always has a tendency to recur after treatment has commenced, and sometimes after it will recur even after it has been cleared for a few weeks or even months, and that is because the perfect breeding conditions for these microorganisms is what is normal for Black hair. So we have to be on a constant vigil.

I can see the shocked look on your faces and hear you ask "Well... then! What exactly can I do to prevent this, and is there any point, if it is going to happen anyway?!!" What I have done over the years, for myself, my daughter, family, friends and clients is adhered to a good hair care routine as described in the wash day chapter, and use products that nourish, moisturise and prevent or inhibit the excessive growth of bad microorganisms. These products are easily absorbed by the scalp and do not sit on the scalp blocking the follicles and pores, preventing the scalp from breathing. This has helped to keep my hair and the hair of everyone who adheres to my advice healthy. This is the same advice that I am giving in this book. I was moved to write this book by all the encouragement from family and friends that more people needed to hear this advice.

Traction-alopecia is also a condition that affects the hair. The appearance of bald patches is called alopecia, and when it is caused by applying too much pressure/ traction to hair it is referred to as traction-alopecia. This is caused by repeatedly pulling the hair tight/ hard (traction) or applying great tension (traction) when placing hair in a hairstyle, especially cornrows on any natural hair and hair braided with extensions. Single braids and the cornrows done for weave-in and wig styles if done inappropriately can also cause traction-alopecia.

When the hair is pulled tight, it puts undue amounts of pressure on the hair root, causing distortion to the follicle, uprooting the hair, cutting off the blood supply and damaging the dermal papilla. When this is regularly done it has a compound of damaging effects to the hair follicle and the dermal papilla. Over time, the hair follicle may go dormant or may eventually die and close off. Once the hair follicle and dermal papilla are dead no hair grows in that area. The condition can be reversed, IF damage is not too far gone and the follicles are not dead. Great care should be taken to stimulate and care for the damaged area and the rest of the hair.

Traction-alopecia is a major problem for Black ladies who wear or have worn braids, cornrows, wigs and weaves for a long time, and other races who normally wear their hair in tight buns. This is because whenever they have had their hair plaited or in a bun, the hair has been plaited or pulled too tight, putting pressure on the hair root. A common misconception is the hair will last longer if you plait it tight. The problem with this is you may come across hairdressers that don't actually know how to plait hair properly. When the technique for plaiting hair is wrong, pressure will be put on the hair root, when that wrong plait is super tight, that pressure has increased tenfold!

If you have traction-alopecia (not alopecia caused by something else) this is down to the improper application-technique of braids or cornrows and tight buns. There will be other factors that increase your risk for traction-alopecia, such as the strength and condition of your hair and hair care routine of your own hair. Your hairdresser or stylist should be able to advise you of the best option for your hair. Please see a reputable hairdresser to help with this problem.

I would like to stress here, that, if the alopecia is caused by an infection or genetic disorder please see a doctor to treat the infection or genetic condition first, as that is the only way the problem will get better, and sometimes you may have to prepare yourself for the possibility that the infections or disorders may have caused irreversible damage.

A hairdresser will only be able to give palliative care to your scalp until the conditions or infections are resolved.

Food also plays a big role in how healthy our hair and scalp is. This is because your hair growth and scalp are nourished by the nutrients that you consume in your food. If your diet is healthy your scalp and hair will be healthy by default, and if your diet is unhealthy, so will be your hair and scalp.

You may want to consume foods that will help boost your hair growth and strengthen your hair. Here are a few foods to help your hair be its best beautiful: oily fish or supplements containing any of the essential omega fatty acids. The higher your omega consumption the better for your hair. The omegas help contribute to the formation of a strong cell membrane. The cell membrane is important because it maintains a strong and properly functioning cell. These cells will do their job most effectively. In the case of our hair, it means our hair will be formed of strong dead keratinized cells that will be hard to damage.

Nuts. They provide trace minerals, plant based protein (which is metabolised better by our body) fatty acids and vitamin D. These are all essential in the production of healthy hair. Green vegetables and brown bread provide trace minerals and vitamin D. Including these foods in an overall healthy diet will boost scalp and hair health by producing strong scalp and hair cells. Strong cells means cells that can easily fight off microorganisms and cells that do not damage easily. So what you eat is really important if you want to have healthy scalp and hair.

Chapter 3

PRODUCTS

Choosing products is one of the single biggest dilemmas for all people, especially those with Afro hair of all different shaped curls. With new products bouncing onto the market in record time, it's no wonder we get confused as to what to use on our hair and scalp. There is so much information out there, good and bad; different products, how to use them, how to make your own etc etc; this is scary and intimidating. I remember when I first went natural, I was freaked out about what I was going to do with my hair and what I needed to put in it. I knew I wanted the products for my hair to be beneficial to me. However, I still felt overwhelmed with the options available. What I did come to realise, sooner rather than later, is that there are a lot of hair products out there that have unnecessary-and-actually-bad-for-your-hair-and-scalp ingredients in them. The task now became to try to find products with ingredients that would nourish, enhance and be beneficial to my scalp and hair.

For me, finding products for myself and my daughter was always a chore. "Will it help? Won't it help?" was always the constant dilemma. Then I started making my own hair products and that dilemma was reduced by about 80%.

How did I start making my own hair products? It was born out of the frustration of not being able to find something to help my daughter's scalp condition, and trying too many products with not-so-good ingredients in them, products that just sat on the scalp blocking it. When my daughter was just over five years old, in the summer of 2003, she came home one day with sand in her hair from her school's sand pit.

Within a week her hair started to fall out (crazy shedding going on). Within two weeks she had a bald spot the size of a two pound coin on her occipital ridge, at the back of her head. (Once the bald spot appeared I stopped sharing combs with her. I went out and bought all new combs for myself). I took her to the doctors and they said the skin looked healthy, so nothing to worry about, but they prescribed me the 'tar' shampoo just to be on the safe side. I had to use this every day. "Have you seen her hair, do you understand that I am Black and we do not, cannot, wash our hair every single day!" I felt like screaming at them. But I didn't. I politely took the prescription and collected the shampoo all the while wondering how I was going to help my daughter, without having to resort to this ridiculousness.

You will understand my dilemma when you read the section on hair wash day.

I tried though. I used to put the shampoo in her dry hair daily and wash it out on the third or fourth day, whichever was permissible. After four weeks I went back to the doctor. By this time the bald spot was nearly the size of my palm, and the hair being shed was about two fists full every time I combed her hair. I was prescribed two more medications to add in with the tar shampoo, and told to wash daily. This time I did say that it was not possible to wash her hair daily but I could do once a week. At this time I still wasn't given any diagnosis for her condition, nor were any tests done to find out what was going on.

Her hair had stopped growing and I was worried that at the rate at which her hair was falling out she'd have no hair left in six months time.

One year, six different diagnoses from six different doctors and a cabinet full of different topical medical applications later, she had multiple bald spots all over her head, with the largest being on her occipital ridge. I could fit the palm of my hand in this space with some room to spare! Bear in mind a five year old's head is not very big in comparison to an adult's palm. To say that I was frustrated was an understatement! By this time her scalp was extremely itchy, tender, puss filled sores all over, with excessive dandruff, and her hair smelled really bad, nearly all the time, apart from the first two days after hair wash day. This was unlike any dandruff I had ever seen, the skin that was coming off her scalp was blood streaked and wafer like pieces that were so thick they would not break away from the hair unless you pulled them out! I had to pull them from her scalp to the tip of the hair strands that were caught in it and off. By this time when I went back to the doctors they would remark "It's not the same problem again, is it?"

You see, as the condition of my daughter's hair was so bad, I was embarrassed for the doctors to see it like that, so I used to always make sure her hair was washed, anything from one to four days before her GP appointment. This is true for many people, embarrassment takes over and we don't present the real problem. We're embarrassed because we don't want anyone to know we have a scalp problem. So we wear wigs, weaves and other things to hide our natural hair, saying "We don't have good hair."

Now it's one thing to be embarrassed and seek resolution, however, it's an entirely different thing to be embarrassed and live with the problem convincing oneself that that is normal, that your hair and scalp just happen to be like that, because as I mentioned before, you may have had the problem from a young age because of sharing combs with family members who had the problem before you. Embarrassment in this case only serves as a detrimental factor in preventing you from seeking treatment. Don't live in silence or undercover, go get help.

In the first six months of back and forth appointments at the GPs they never really saw the full extent of her hair condition. Why was I embarrassed? I don't know. I guess on some level, I didn't want anyone thinking I was neglecting my daughter. The last straw came when the diagnosis I got from the last doctor was "I think it could be fleas, maybe your place needs to be fumigated. That's probably why it's spreading to you." The reason she said this was, whenever I was plaiting my daughter's hair, as she would be sitting on a stool between my legs as I combed her hair, the dandruff would fall on my thighs and by the next morning I would notice that all the hair where the dandruff had fallen on me had died and I'd have multiple bald spots all over my thighs. I had told her this, and instead of testing she decided to tell me that I wasn't cleaning my house properly or practicing good hygiene for my daughter.

Needless to say I went home absolutely fuming, got out my daughter's baby medical book, where I had documented every single diagnosis and prescribed medication. I decided to make another appointment and confront them with my records. Next day I rang and asked to make an appointment with the senior GP at the surgery, who happened to be our GP as well. His next availability was a week later. I took it. When the day came I was petrified, but I did it anyway. When I confronted him with my evidence he had no option but to refer me to Kingston Hospital's Dermatology department urgently.

We were seen within two weeks. After blood tests, hair scrapings, pulling out my baby's hair from the hair follicle to have the root intact, and a scalp sample later (that's scary, they used something like a weirdly shaped nail clipper and pinched a bit of the skin off from one of the bald spots), it turned out that she had a fungal infection in her hair follicles. Unfortunately because it had taken a year for me to force them to test her, the fungus was now in her bloodstream and would have to be treated from there, before her scalp would show any sign of improvement.

Medicines were ordered as the hospital did not stock that drug. It was rarely used on children and was sparingly given to adults. They told me that it was likely the infection would come back after the dose was finished but she could not be re-prescribed these meds for another ten years! Yup you read right, ten years... that's how strong these meds are and it had to be completely out of your system, and your system given time to heal before you could have them again. No topical ones were given as doctors said it had to be cured from her blood first, but I was told to continue with what I already had at home from previous prescriptions. Medication arrived within a week and I started giving it to her straight away.

Within a week her hair started to grow back! The bad smell reduced and the sores went away.

We were away in the USA for first three weeks when the medication kicked in. By the time we came back to the UK, her hair had grown about an inch in every bald spot. Dandruff had reduced, and the smell was more or less gone, but came back with a vengeance every time she sweated in her hair. Which was actually VERY often, because I have never met anyone with more hair per square inch of scalp, and I have seen and touched many many scalps.

Whilst away I had vowed to find alternative topical applications that would help her scalp seeing as what I had already wasn't working. Upon arrival at home, I threw away every hair product that I had had for her, apart from the 'tar' shampoo and the conditioner I was using for her at the time. I bought a big bottle of extra virgin olive oil and that was it. Three products for her hair, done! Medication was done in three weeks and I wanted to make sure I did everything in my power to prevent a recurrence and if it so did return it would not be as devastating as it was previously.

This was when my research into hair and scalp health began in earnest. I read up on everything I could and watched YouTube videos. I was at a loss of how to improve her hair and scalp health and still keep it fungus free. I became one of those moms who told my child on a daily basis, "Do not let your hair or head touch anyone else's or let them touch your hair under any circumstances, this includes adults too, make sure you wash your hands before you touch your own hair. No Touching your hair or scalp, by you or ANYONE period!" Petrified of what might happen if the fungus came back. Three months in and I added Asian jasmine hair oil to her hair regime. For the next five years I continued with this simple hair care regime. However, I could tell her hair was lacking. It wasn't the best it could be but it was fungus free, growing and mildly healthy, and I was determined to keep it that way.

It wasn't until I started my training as an Aromatherapist that this path was suddenly enlightened for me. I finally had a way of keeping her scalp and hair healthy and fungus free. The experimentation began. I worked my way through carefully crafted essential oil synergies. Synergy after synergy, in all manner of different base combinations until I came up with one that made both her and my hair and scalp healthy and kept the fungus away.

This was my first product, and I named it "*Ommi's Beauty Hair Butter.*" This product we used as a family. I even shipped some to my brothers in America and they loved it. I also then looked at making my own oil mix as I discovered that the Asian jasmine oil had more mineral oil in it than the beneficial jasmine oil. I made my own hair oil, after researching different oils and their beneficial properties through trial and error, and came up with the best possible combination, for maximum results. This is "*Ommi's Beauty Liquid Gold Hair Oil*." I have never bought hair butter, oil or cream product from the shops since. I used this combination on my daughter's hair and her hair took off, to the point that people used to ask me if her hair was real! I used these products myself and also started using them on my clients with great results.

But in 2011 the fungus struck back! I took her to the doctors straight away, explaining our history with this. They understood but still couldn't do anything about it at the moment, as it was only eight years since she last had the previous medication. I was told to come back in two years time if the problem still persisted, and in the meantime was prescribed all the same topical medical applications that didn't really work last time round. I went away this time with the determination that I was going to make something that would keep this fungus in check once and for all! So the research began, and after some trial and error, "Ommi's Beauty Hairssential Oil" was born. This is a concentration of six different essential oils that have antifungal and hair growth stimulating properties amongst a host of others, in nourishing base oil. So not only does it keep your scalp and hair free from microorganisms, it also boosts your hair growth.

This I used on my daughter's scalp, and it kept the fungus at bay. After two years of not being treated at the source, I was slowly losing the battle. The more the fungus built up in her bloodstream the worse her scalp got. This is one of the reasons why I stress in the previous chapter that you need to treat any problem at the source before any topical application can work to prevent it. Then in 2013 we were able to get the antifungal prescription and we have since been able to keep her hair and scalp healthy with just "*Ommi's Beauty Hair Products*".

The range now consists of a "Nourishing Hair Cream" as well, and that came into being when a couple of clients mentioned that the butter was too heavy for their hair. This cream is lighter than the butter, and so full of natural goodness and lots of moisture that I like to think of it as 'crack' for the hair, because, it makes your hair feel and look like it's as high as a kite. It packs a power punch of nourishing butters and oils and essential moisture, all rolled into one handy product.

If you are going to try any of *Ommi's Beauty products* this should be your item. I readjusted the butter mix so it would complement the hair cream, so the butter is now a *sealing butter*. The full range of products available at *Ommi's Beauty* is *Ommi's Beauty Nourishing Hair Cream, Liquid Gold Hair Oil,*

Sealing Hair Butter and Hairssential Hair Growth Stimulating Oil. They are all organic, the mixtures are well balanced and each ingredient and its percentage is carefully chosen to work in a synergy to help your hair be its best beautiful.

I concentrated on these four, and looked elsewhere to source the rest seeing as I could not make all the hair products my hair would ever need. Through trial and error, and by process of elimination, I settled upon Arbonne International products. Their products are all plant based and vegan certified and make my family's hair look and feel amazing. In making my products I still wanted to give back to the community, so all my ingredients are reasonably sourced and fairly traded, and Arbonne reflected this as well.

So what do products do? First we have to ask, "What does our hair need?" This question is what should drive our product selection. Generally, for all races, the hair and scalp needs moisture, which equals water and oils or butters, which impart lipids (organic compounds that are fatty acids or their derivatives, these include natural oils and natural butters) to the hair shaft, the hair follicles and the surrounding skin as nutrition and nourishment. These natural oils and natural butters can be used as a sealant, which is normally a heavier oil or butter to seal all that goodness into the hair shaft, preventing moisture and nutrition loss. Products need to be such that they do not block or inhibit the life cycle of the hair and skin cells.

Your products need to be easily absorbed into the hair shaft, follicles and skin. They need to be readily utilised by your dermal papilla and skin cells for the benefit of your hair and scalp. They should not create a barrier on the scalp. If they do, they will drastically reduce the rate of desquamation (the process by which our dead skin cells are shed) of the cells of the scalp, which could lead to all sorts of problems and dead skin cell build up.

Products that are beneficial to your hair and scalp make your hair feel soft, moisturised, supple and smooth. Hair has a healthy glow and shine to it. Your scalp will feel clean at all times, with relatively no build-up, it will be well moisturised with little to no dandruff.   Any products that do not do this for your scalp and hair are best left alone. You will know if your product is working well for you by the lack of build-up in your hair and on your scalp. Your hair will be easily cleaned with no feeling of greasy gunk on your scalp.

When your products don't work for you, you will see a buildup of dead skin cells (excessive dandruff), build-up of products on hair and scalp causing hair to have white flaky residue all over and scalp to be itchy with greasy-like buildup that gets trapped under nails. This stops your skin cells from desquamating naturally. Products may also change the ph of your scalp which can sometimes produce a bad smell. If a product is causing any of the above, please stop using it. No matter how much it cost you to buy it, stop using it immediately.

If you want to finish it to get your money's worth, you may end up causing more damage to your hair and scalp over time, as anything we use on our hair and scalp has a cumulative effect, whether good or bad. You could be doing yourself more harm than good by carrying on using a product that doesn't work for you.

It took me awhile to get into this habit, as like you all, I felt I was wasting my money if I didn't use it all up. However, it actually cost me more financially and time wise, every time I did this, to eventually repair the damage done by using the wrong products for my hair.

What should we be looking for? There are oils, lotions, creams, butters, leave-in conditioners, hair serum, and many many more. Lighter oils and lotions should be used on low porosity hair. This is because the molecules of lighter oils and lotions are smaller in size and as such are able to penetrate into the hair shaft between the tightly packed cuticles of low porosity hair. A light cream or mousse is ideal to use as well

Heavier oils, creams and butters can be used on normal to high porosity hair. This is because their molecules are larger, but due to the slightly larger gaps in the cuticles of normal to high porosity hair, the larger molecules are able to pass through.

Leave-in conditioners can be used on all hair types. There are lotion types and liquid types, and you need to find out what works best for your hair and use it.

Hair needs water to keep it moisturized as well as the above. If you can douse your hair with water, or wash your hair, before applying any of the above that would help your hair.

For non afro hair, you will want to apply any oils, creams or butters before washing your hair. Douse hair with water, apply oils, creams or butters, from root to tip and all over scalp. Pile hair on top of head, cover with a plastic cap and leave for a minimum of 30min. Longer than that is up to you but better for your hair. Anything up to 2hrs is great.

However please don't just apply the oil and then sit twiddling your thumbs. You can use that time to catch up on housework, paperwork, TV or media time, or whatever you want to do.

Please bear in mind, for low porosity hair you will need to leave the product on longer as the molecules of the product need to work their way under the cuticle and into the hair shaft, and when the gaps are small this will take time.

Once you are done with the oils, apply conditioner all over hair, cover with plastic cap and leave for another 30min. Dampen with water, lather conditioner and rinse out. Try and get a good lather going by adding water to hair little by little. You then wash hair with a shampoo, condition hair and style as normal.

Treatment

Treatments are an injection of power packed shots for hair. You have steam, heat, oils and masks. They deliver a concentrated infusion of nutrition, strengthening and or cleansing properties to hair and the scalp.

Steam and heat must never be used just on their own, they must always follow an application of a deep conditioner or oil. The reason being, steam and heat will open up the hair cuticles and cause all the moisture in the hair to evaporate, severely drying out the hair.

The deep conditioning and nourishing treatments should be left on for a minimum of 30 minutes but no longer than an hour. However, longer is not going to harm your hair. I must admit I have left my deep conditioning treatment on sometimes a 'wee' bit longer, when I've got stuck doing something.

Nutrition treatments are treatments that deliver nourishing goodness to hair and scalp, delivering ingredients that moisturise, soften hair and help it to grow. These will include deep conditioning treatments, natural food and herbal hair masks, and oils or butters masks.

Strengthening treatments are the ones that deliver ingredients that harden the keratinized cells of the hair, fill in the gaps in the hair shaft caused by damage, and help create stronger bonds between the cells of the hair. These treatments help to retain length by preventing breakage and split ends. They also fill in the gaps in the cuticle of damaged hair by bonding to the protein in the hair cells and bonding to each other.

In the anatomy and physiology section, we talked about how hair cannot heal or repair itself, but can be repaired by putting a bandage over the damage. Well, your strengthening treatments are your bandage. So, if your hair has a lot of damage you want to have these on a regular basis until new healthy hair grows through. A word of advice here, please please please, always follow a strengthening treatment with conditioning or deep conditioning after.

This is because the strengthening treatment will make your hair feel very wiry and coarse, and can lead to dryness and breakage (the very thing we are trying to prevent) if not properly moisturised after. Your hair is a 'crisp' here and you want it to be a 'slice of potato'. The strengthening treatments should be left on hair for a minimum of 30 minutes, but no longer than 45 minutes. Really important, as any longer will produce the 'crisp' effect.

Strengthening treatments include your protein treatments, ayurvedic treatments, ayurvedic hair teas, rice water rinses, clays and herbal masks.

Rice water rinses I have found incredible useful in reducing the shedding of my hair. The trace minerals that are found in raw rice and the fermentation process are what help impart such benefits to the hair and scalp. Rice water rinses help strengthen and anchor your hair root, preventing excess shedding. It also helps to strengthen hair shaft and improve elasticity, reducing breakage, thus increasing length. Each portion of rice used should be mixed with five times the amount of water (1cup rice to 5cups water) and be left for at least 24hrs (48hrs is ideal) at room temperature to ferment.

The rice is then strained from the water when it is ready for use. The fermented rice water is used to rinse the hair, from scalp to tip of hair. I know fermented rice water sounds yucky to put on your hair, but it doesn't smell bad, just ricey, however, if you leave it longer than two days it does smell rank (I know), so please don't use that on your scalp. Throw it away and start again. This rinse can be done once every two weeks before deep conditioning, and left on for 10 minutes to a maximum of 30 minutes. Apply deep conditioner to scalp and hair without rinsing the rice water out. Leave the mixture on hair for 30 minutes or 10 minutes with a heat cap. Rinse out and style as normal.

Cleansing treatments are treatments that clean out build up of hair products and dead skin cells from the hair, hair follicles and scalp. These are important to aid desquamation and keep your hair and scalp renewed. These include your clay, herbal, ayurvedic, natural food masks and rinses. Cleansing treatments should be left on hair for a minimum of 30 minutes, but no longer than 45 minutes. Any longer and it will produce the 'crisp' effect.

After a strengthening or cleansing treatment, you need to follow with a rich deep conditioning one. You can supercharge your deep conditioner with the recipe at the end of this chapter. That should be left on for a minimum of 30 minutes, but 45 minutes to an hour is ideal. If you use a steamer or a heat cap with any of these treatments cut the minimum time down to half! For best results, always follow a cleansing or strengthening treatment with a nourishing treatment, which only needs to be left on for 15 to 30 minutes, then follow that with a deep conditioner. All these treatment times can be cut down to a third of the time if a heat cap (steam or dry) is used. I would advise against using a heat cap all the time, as this can lead to over processing. Use only when you are in an awful hurry.

How do you put all this into your hair care routine?

Always deep-condition whenever you wash and condition your hair. Nourishing treatments should be done every 2 to 3 weeks, and a strengthening treatment should be done every 4 to 6 weeks. If you over do the strengthening treatments, hair can become brittle and dry. Overdoing the cleansing treatment will produce dryness and increase porosity. Cleansing treatments should only be done every 3 to 4 months. As the treatments are so deep-cleansing they can have a stripping and drying effect on the hair, they should always be followed with a nourishing treatment and then conditioner, or at the very least a deep conditioner. This you can weave into your hair care routine when the time arrives, whenever you feel your hair needs a good clean-out.

If you are new to starting on a healthy hair care routine with good products that work for your hair, I would recommend you do a cleansing treatment first, to get rid of all the old stuff and start on a blank canvas. This makes sure that your new-good-for-your hair-and-scalp products have no resistance or interference from buildup of old products and dead skin cells.

For Chemically processed hair

A strengthening treatment should ideally be done 7 to 10 days after any chemical processing (perming, straightening, colouring). This gives the hair a rest period after the processing but not enough time to start to get dry and brittle. An ayurvedic treatment is especially good for this time, and should be followed by a deep conditioning treatment, always.

Then 2 weeks after your ayurvedic, a protein treatment would be ideal, and should also always be followed by a deep conditioning treatment for best results.

Then 2 weeks after your protein treatment a deep conditioning treatment.

2 weeks after that, another deep conditioning treatment. This should then bring you full cycle to your next chemical processing appointment, which is about every 6 minimum to 8 maximum weeks apart.

So ideally, in between your chemical processing, straightening, colouring or curling treatments, you should have one strengthening treatment, one protein treatment, and two deep conditioning treatments, in that order, ideally spaced about two weeks apart.

Naturally Straight or Curly Hair that is coloured

People with these hair types may follow the above hair strengthening and nourishing routine, however, you may wish to space the treatments out to a 12 week interval or space them out between your haircut or your regular salon visits.

If you visit the salon quite regularly, then you might want to space the treatments above over 3 to 4 maybe even 5 salon visits. It all depends on the frequency of your visits and the condition of your hair.

For bleached hair, you may want to keep your treatments within a 6 to 8 week period. For coloured hair, you may want to space your treatments within a 10 to 12 week period, as colouring also has a milder-than-bleaching weakening effect on the hair.

Cleansing Hair Mask

3 tbs of rhassoul cleansing clay

1 tbs of rose petal powder

1½ tbs of shikakai powder

5 tbs aloe juice

100 ml of your favourite conditioner *(mine is Arbonne's Nourishing Daily Conditioner)*

Mix the powders together, then add aloe juice, and slowly add water to make into a paste. Apply to hair as part of your hair care routine following the above guidelines.

Nourishing Hair Mask

1 egg yolk

1 avocado

2 tbs of natural yoghurt

2 tbs of olive oil

2 tbs of honey

2½ tbs of palm oil (may substitute with castor oil)

Place all in a NutriBullet and blitz. Apply to hair as part of your hair care routine following the above guidelines.

Strengthening / Protein Hair Mask

2 tbs of natural yoghurt

1 large banana or 2 small ones

1 tbs of honey

1 egg (or just the egg white for halving the recipe)

3 tbs of coconut oil

2 tbs of sesame seed oil

Place all in a NutriBullet and blitz. Apply to hair as part of your hair care routine following the above guidelines.

Supercharge your deep conditioner

100 ml of your favourite conditioner *(mine is Arbonne's Hair Revitalising Masque)*

1½ tbs of castor oil

½ tbs of avocado oil

½ tbs sesame seed oil

10 drops of ginger essential oil

10 drops of bergamot essential oil

Find a suitable jar or bowl that you can mix the ingredients in and use them from. I like to use empty jam or honey jars for myself and family, and for my clients I mix the ingredients in my hair colouring bowl. Put the deep conditioner into the container first, then add the oils and essential oils. Mix thoroughly and apply to hair as part of your hair care routine following the above guidelines.

DIY leave-in conditioner

1 tbs of your favourite conditioner *(mine is Arbonne's Nourishing Daily Conditioner)*

2.5ml of glycerin

2.5ml of avocado oil

5ml of castor oil

10ml of aloe juice

5 drops of ginger essential oil

5 drops of ylang-ylang essential oil

Place conditioner, glycerin and oils into a 250 ml spray bottle. Shake until well mixed. Add the essential oils and aloe juice and shake until mixed. Now slowly top up with water, mixing as you do so, to fill the bottle up to 250 ml. This will last you about 2 to 3 weeks depending on length and thickness of hair and how often you use your leave-in. You can use ionised, bottled or boiled water to make it last even longer and keep the sterility of the product. For naturally straight or curly hair you may want to omit the oils completely or use lighter oils like jojoba and argan, and might also need to use in smaller quantities.

Depending on the length and thickness of your hair please either double up on the ingredients for longer and or thicker hair, or halve them for finer and or shorter hair. If you have any allergies to any of the ingredients listed, please please swap them for ones that you are not allergic to.

You can buy all the specialist ingredients in these above mixes from the Akoma website. I get all my ingredients from them. I like the fact that all the products are responsibly sourced and most are Fairly Traded. I have used them now for many years as their products are always of a superior quality.

Curly Proverbz is a YouTube vlogger that gives good information on ayurvedic hair treatments and hair teas. Do look at her videos for recipes and how to use and make lots of different ayurvedic treatments.

Naptural85 is another YouTube vlogger that gives manageable hair styles and hair treatments and product recommendations for Black hair.

These are my two favourite YouTubers, I find their content beneficial to all hair types generally, but especially for Black hair.

Chapter 4

Healthy Hair Practices

H
air Wash Day!

Arrrrrrrrrggg............ , hands on the head and thinking "good Lord, is it that time already?"

This is the reaction of most Black women when it comes to washing their hair or their children's hair. I have been told by moms of curly haired children of mixed parentage that they have a similar reaction. I know it was certainly mine, for a very long time and definitely for the most part of my daughter's childhood. Not anymore.

I used to dread 'hair wash day', because it would take the whole day, literally, with tears and tantrums from my daughter, my scalp feeling 'sour' (sore or tender), and me being absolutely exhausted at the end of it, falling into bed and thinking, "thank God I only have to do this every 4 weeks. I remember thinking every time "there has got to be an easier way to do this!" But without fail, in 4 weeks time hair wash day would come round and be exactly the same. This is because I didn't know any better. So I did what I was familiar with, even though I knew, in my heart of hearts, there just had to be a better way, I hadn't found it yet. I carried on as 'normal' until I went natural (stopped all chemical processing) with my hair. This was my pivot point.

I was getting busier with work, my daughter's hair was waist length, and 'hair wash day' was a whole day dedicated to washing her hair alone. No time to do mine. I remember we always had take-away food, and would break for lunch and dinner. Sometimes we'd get done just before dinner, and that would be a great day. Bed straight after, poor child was absolutely shattered! That was exactly how I grew up with 'hair wash day'.

As we got older we would take over the job of washing our own hair and then mom or older girls in the house would plait the hair, saving everyone a job. However, nobody really knew how to wash their hair to avoid creating a mass of tangles; it was always scary going to have your hair plaited after you had washed it, as the detangling was not done gently! I remember thinking "I can't wait for her to be big enough to wash her own hair, that way I could have a rest and then just plait it. This is what traditionally happened in Liberian households.

My problem was my daughter's hair was too long for her to handle, as she had never handled it during washing before. This is what we learned when the time came and I started to wean her off my hair care time. At first she couldn't even manage to comb her hair thoroughly as it was so very thick and long. The first few washes she did herself were a total disaster! I had to rewash her hair straight after. Her scalp and hair weren't clean. This made 'hair wash day' twice as long. On a few occasions 'hair wash day' spanned two days! And because she had the scalp fungal problem, it was paramount that her hair was clean on hair wash day.

Thankfully, over time I came to realise that there is a better way. If I had known then, what I know now... hair wash day would have been a whole different story!

So why is 'hair wash day' a problem in so many households? Have we been doing it wrong all these years? Generation after generation this is passed down, and yet we have a problem. We have a problem with growth, length and retention. How does washing your hair affect these? Let me explain. When we don't wash our hair properly, we cause so much trauma to our hair and scalp, that it is easier for our hair to be pulled out. This affects retention, breaks off length, and stunts growth.

How often should we wash our hair and why?

Well... for generation after generation, from household to household, amongst Africans, Afro-American, Afro-Caribbean and the kinky curly afro population in general, because of the hair styles we wear, we tend to wash our hair once in 4 to 12 weeks! I have known people who have gone much much longer, and believe you me when I say, "You do not want to be around when they open their hair!" I remember a friend once remarking "it seems like something has crawled up and died in there!" It is only in the last couple of years, since the natural hair movement has taken its hold, that the question of "how often should we wash our hair?" has come into play. So... how often should we do the do? What is too much, too little or just right?

Kinky, curly, afro hair should be washed once every 7 to 10 days. For other hair types it is best washed once every 3 to 7 days. However, based on the different types of hairstyles people wear this might not be possible. As you will read below, it is best to wash your hair when it's not all braided or tied up, in any way, shape or form. The reason we wash our hair is because our hair produces sebum, to moisturise scalp and hair and seal hair cuticle. Over time, this can build up on hair and scalp. For straighter hair types this is very true. However, for kinky, curly, afro hair types the sebum mostly builds up on the scalp and on about only a 5th or 6th of the actual hair shaft, the bit closest to the scalp.

This is due to the curl of the hair. The curl lifts the hair up and away from the scalp, and since sebum travels by osmosis and gravity, it's quite hard to get the sebum to the hair's end that's pointing upwards. There's also a build up of products on our hair, and this is for all hair types. However, the types of products used determines just how much (or how bad) a build up you have on your hair and scalp, as mentioned in the 'products' chapter of this book. If we use products that are petroleum based or have a lot of synthetic ingredients in them, they sit on our scalp and hair without penetrating to provide nourishment, and trap dead skin cells, bacteria and or fungi to our scalp, and do not allow the scalp to breathe.

Breathing of the scalp is the passing in and out of substances in our scalp, for the cells in your scalp and hair to be able to utilise the topical nourishment that you provide for them (this is breathing in), and your scalp to be able to secrete sebum and excrete sweat (this is breathing out), to form the acid mantle to protect your scalp and hair from microorganisms. Synthetic ingredients also get absorbed into our scalp. We have to remember that, at all times, our skin can absorb up to 60% of what is placed on it, so if you do not want it in your bloodstream do not put it on your skin, and this includes hair care products. Good healthy products have the advantage of having molecules small enough to enter into our scalp and hair with ease; they also impart topical nourishment to our scalp and hair, helping them to grow healthily. This is a healthy balance.

We want products that pass through easily as well as allow the scalp to breathe. In this way when it comes to wash day you won't have a buildup of products, dead skin cells, bacteria etc to wash away. The less build up on your hair and scalp the easier it will be to wash your hair, and the quicker your hair will get clean. What this means is, you will need less cleaning products for your hair, less soapy products too.

So how are we supposed to wash our hair?

Well the purpose of washing the hair is to get it clean and add moisture, so it really doesn't matter what you use, as long as the end result is a clean head of hair that is well moisturized. It is cleaning the build up of products and pollution from one's hair.

BUT... what is really important is what you do before you wash and after you wash hair to MINIMISE tangling! Therein lies the crux of the matter for Black hair. This is actually a universal problem, but with other races hair, the before and after is much less tenuous. The principle applies to all: minimise tangling so that styling is a breeze.

So what do we do before? Pre-poo. Pre-poo is short for pre-shampoo. What is this and how do you do it? The purpose of this is to smooth the cuticles on the hair shaft to make the process of detangling easier and much less stressful on the hair shaft and hair root, thus reducing damage and breakage to the hair. This is done using oils and or butters to coat the hair from root to tip, liberally. Now, non afro hair may not require as much oils and or butters. Use what your hair needs and works well with your hair, creating shine, slippage and softening. Always start with very little and work up from there.

You will know you have enough on your hair when your hair strands slide easily past one another. Best not to use a water-based product for pre-poo, as water softens and causes shrinkage to the hair. It is best to use very nourishing oils or butters for this process, as you want to always be imparting nutrients to your hair. You can keep the oils and or butters from your pre-poo on your head for about 5min to overnight.

I normally leave mine in overnight. When you are pre-pooing after taking out extensions, you will have some or a lot of fluff around the base of each plait (cornrow or single braid), depending on the length of time you kept the extensions in. There will be more matting in this area too. You want to make sure you get rid of all of the fluff that you can. Start by using your fingers, and when you can't get anymore off, use a very soft baby brush, the kind that is used on newborns hair, and brush the remaining fluff.

Only leave what you absolutely cannot get off. The reason this is important is the fluff will cause undue amount of knots in your hair that you won't be able to undo and will have to cut out. You also get fluff if you keep one hairstyle in too long. Always have a scissors with you when pre-pooing and detangling. This is for cutting out any knots. It is better for your hair strands for the knots to be cut out than to be ripped out, which is what combing knots out will do.

Detangling

The reason we get tangles is because our hair strands wrap around each other and all the shed hair is wrapped around the hair strands that are still attached to our heads.

After pre-poo you should move straight into your detangling. You would use your fingers at this stage. For those of you who only do finger detangling then you would use your fingers throughout your hair washing. For me, I do like to get a comb on my scalp and running through my hair, but that comes later.

The reason we don't use combs at this stage is because the comb WILL put too much strain on the dry hair strands and cause damage and breakage. This is because we have just sealed the hair shaft, giving it strength, thereby making it less pliable to the rigorous manipulation the combing through will cause. Now my suggestion here would be, don't try and get your whole hair done at once, but work in portions, manageable portions for you and your hair.

As you go through the portions you want to be pulling the hair apart, and using your fingers to pull out any hairs that have shed and are just sitting there. Use your fingers to comb through each portion of hair. If your fingers don't run smoothly through or you come across any knots, add more oil or butter to the area and work it into the tangled area and gently work the knot loose and the dead hair out.

If you come across any knots that are just too tight to be undone, please don't rip your hair strands apart trying to take it out; and definitely do not pull the knot out of your hair. Get a pair of small scissors and cut the knot out. Cut all the hairs that are attached to the knot close to the knot until it is free. Cutting it out keep the cuticles sealed and creates straight edges on the hair; whilst ripping apart or pulling it out not only hurts your scalp as you are putting so much tension on the hair root, but it frays the edge of the hair strand which leads to unsealed cuticles and split ends.

When you have thoroughly worked through a portion and you are satisfied that you have dealt with all knots, two-finger twist or plait that portion back up.

Keep working until you have completed your whole head of hair. The reason you plait all the portions back up is to make sure they do not re-tangle. Left to their own devices, especially for Afro hair, your hairs will continually hug, lie on top of and wrap around each other, creating a constant flow of knots. You can move straight on to washing your hair or you can leave the oil and or butters in a little longer, up to overnight.

I normally leave mine in overnight, so I pre-poo and detangle my hair before I go to bed. If you are leaving your oils/butters in, you will need to cover your hair with a plastic shower cap. If sleeping in it you might want to use a soft plastic shower cap, so you do not hear it as you move about in bed. Believe me I know. It keeps waking you up! If going to bed or out of the house with your pre-pooed detangled hair, you might want to wear a scarf on your head. Aside from keeping in all the heat from your head and helping the oils/butters penetrate deeper into your hair shaft and hair follicle, a scarf serves as a fashion item or sleep aid. Who needs to know you are pre-pooing your hair under your scarf! I've done it many times :)

After this you can then move on to washing the hair, whichever way you wash your hair.

If you shampoo wash, my suggestion would be, you apply your shampoo to your dry portioned hair, still in their twist or plaits. Once shampoo is applied to the twisted or plaited portions, you then wet the hair. Lather up in your portions, using your fingertips to massage the scalp only, in each portion, paying special care not to place too much stress on the hair strands on the outer edge of each portion. If too much stress is placed on these areas this is what causes breakages and damage within your head of hair. When you massage it is best to do so in the direction your hair is lying in, to go against, will cause stress. The larger the portions the less stress is caused, and the smaller the portion the more stress caused. This is because, in the larger portion, you have more room to massage and maneuver underneath where the plait or twist begins.

This is why it is not good to wash your hair when it is plaited small, with or without extensions. Ever wonder why people who braid their hair, especially with extensions, have longish hair that always tapers to a very thin tip when plaited and also looks very thin ¼ or a ⅓ of the way from the tip? This is because of the damage caused by washing the hair with the plaits or extensions in. It makes the hair break off at the base, around each plait.

Thus these people's hair is always comprised of more hairs that are all different lengths, with the longest being the least. Their hair looks and feels thickest from the root to halfway up. To avoid this sort of damage it is best to remove the small plaits before washing your hair. Once the scalp is massaged and feels clean to you, then gently work the shampoo into the length of the hair and rinse.

Benefit of shampoo washing your hair is it takes out all the dirt without too much of an effort. The downside of this is; because it cleans so deeply so quickly it opens the hair cuticle and it strips the hair of all oils and nutrients. Opening the cuticles makes the hair tangle more, and harder to detangle, thus making the detangling process after washing much longer, especially if you don't wash your hair in portions.

However, if you use shampoos with gentler cleansing ingredients/soaps, or soap-free shampoos, you won't have the stripping or opening of cuticle effect, which is much better for your hair. So you can still use shampoos, just use a mild and or soap-free one. May I add a word of warning here: never ever comb through or attempt to detangle your hair with shampoo in it. If you try to do this, this will not be easy and it will greatly damage your hair. When the cuticles of the hair shaft are already open and the hair shaft is stripped, the hair is more susceptible to damage and breakage. To think that when I was a kid, combing your hair through with the shampoo in it was considered the first step in the detangling process!

My memory tells me this step was always the longest and was ALWAYS the most painful. When the older girls in the house did your hair they didn't care how much pain you were in. They just pulled and pulled to make sure there were no knots. Partly because of time, if your hair wasn't done before your mom came home they would be in trouble, and depending on how many of you there were, time was of the essence. It was also the older girls' way of getting back at you for any annoying thing you had done to them during the week. I remember my hair being done one time, and me going "awh... that hurts" and my older cousin responding with something along the lines "well best remember that next time you go reporting me to Mommie." Hahaha... this makes me laugh so hard. The circle of life is in everything.

If you co-wash, which is short for conditioner wash, you can then go ahead and co-wash your hair after pre-poo and detangling. I now co-wash my hair, and have done so exclusively since about halfway through 2012. I remembered co-washing my hair in Liberia, after being there for 2 weeks. And to be honest I was skeptical as to whether my hair would come up clean as it normally did in the UK. Liberia can be dusty, with this kind of brownish red dust that clings to everything! Coupled with the constant heat, around 23°C every day, making my scalp sweat, I knew my hair would be very dirty, and I wasn't sure my co-washing would be up to the task. I had a mild shampoo at the ready. Suffice it to say my co-wash did the job and did it splendidly! Didn't need the shampoo at all!

To co-wash you apply your conditioner to your detangled portions of hair. Make sure your hair is dry when you do this. Work with one portion at a time. Open the portion of hair and apply the conditioner, working it from root to tip. Once you have enough on, you then apply some water to the portion of hair, to saponify your conditioner. You want to work this into your scalp and hair, massaging your scalp to lift the dirt. You will know you have enough on when your hair stops absorbing the conditioner. For those of you with porous hair your hair will absorb more conditioner. Over time this will change. As you start to follow good practices, your hair will become less porous.

Once you have applied the water over the conditioner to the portion of hair and worked it into your hair and scalp, now is when you would take your comb and comb through the portion of hair until your hair is knot free. If you don't use a comb in your hair, use your fingers or whatever you normally use and go through the portion of hair until it is knot free. Then plait or twist the portion back up and move onto the next portion and repeat the process. Do this until your whole head of hair is done. Once all your hair is done, cover with a shower cap and leave for 10 to 30 minutes. This is where you carry on doing something else, cleaning, reading a book, start preparing food, etc. Use your time wisely. If your hair is very dirty, or hasn't been washed for 2 weeks or more, leave it on for 30 minutes. If this is your weekly wash, 5 to 10 minutes is enough.

When you co-wash you have a gentler cleansing to your hair and moisture infusion for hair and scalp gets a kick start.

The down side of this type of wash is, if you use heavy synthetic unhealthy products, the conditioner will have a hard time lifting these off your hair. Co-washing also helps to make combing the hair through much easier in the whole hair wash process. After your 5 to 30 minutes period, rinse the hair out. You can do this with the portions in your hair or take them out and really give your scalp a good scratching while rinsing out. And I do love a good scratching on my scalp when I wash, so I take my twists out put a little bit of water on my hair and lather up the conditioner, and scratch my scalp clean to my satisfaction. What's best to remember here is, never scratch your hair out when it's in portions of any kind, as this will damage your hair.

If your hair isn't as clean as you'd like, repeat the process above and leave on for 10 minutes. If you have opened your hair to scratch it out, re-apply the conditioner to the whole hair as is, comb through thoroughly and plait into 1, 2, or 3 plaits, or however many your hair can manage, cover and leave for 10 minutes. If you have been using better-for-your-hair products, your hair will be clean the first time round.

After shampooing or co-washing, next step is to condition. Yes, you will still condition even if you co-wash, as that first step is the cleansing rather than the conditioning bit.

If you have shampooed your hair, you would have done this in your portions, right? Good. Now apply the conditioner to each portion, comb through each individual portion and replait or retwist. Carry on as such until you have conditioned your whole hair. Cover your hair with a plastic shower cap and leave for 10 to 20 minutes. Rinse off in portions. If this is your last step definitely do not undo your portions. However, if you are going to deep condition then you may or may not undo your portions, rinse off and apply deep conditioner, comb through and replait or retwist. However, my recommendation would be to keep your hair in plaited or twisted portions and apply your deep conditioner to hair portion by portion and keep them in portions to rinse out.

Deep Conditioning, why is this Important?

Deep conditioning is very essential for anyone who wants healthy hair and scalp, especially for those who want to grow long hair, regardless of race, skin colour or hair type. It also improves the health of your hair and scalp. It delivers important moisture (water) to the hair, with oils and or butters to nourish scalp and hair. Our hair is strengthened by the amount of nutrients supplied to it topically and internally (diet), and the amount of moisture keeping it supple. The nourishment goes towards improving the medulla and cortex of the hair. The moisture keeps the hair flexible, so that it avoids breakage and damage. Let me give you an example. I want you think of your hair as fresh potato or potato crisp.

Well moisturized hair will be a very thin slice of fresh potato and damaged dry hair will be one slice of crisp. Which one of those do you think you are able to move about without breaking? The slice of fresh potato will move about freely until a point. If you put too much pressure on the slice of potato, it breaks. On the other hand, the slice of potato crisp is immovable and any attempt at manipulation results in breakage. Your hair is exactly the same.

Well moisturized hair gives room for normal manipulation (combing, finger detangling) and styling (the 'slice of fresh potato effect'), and dry hair breaks easily under very little pressure (the 'crisp effect'). A deep conditioning treatment will improve your hair regardless of hair type. This should be done at least once every 2 weeks. For those of your trying to get length, a deep conditioning treatment should be done every week or every time you wash your hair.

If we always remember the slice of potato and crisp analogy, we will always remember to style our hair under the right conditions and improve how well we keep our hair moisturized. The oils in the deep conditioner also help the cuticles on the hair shaft to lie flat and seal very well, creating a near watertight barrier, thus sealing in the moisture in the hair shaft, this also makes the hair look shiny, as the cuticles lying flat and sealed create a reflective surface.

You can buy a specific deep conditioning product or you can supercharge your normal conditioner by adding oils and or butters to it to make it a nourishing deep conditioner. See recipe in products chapter on how to make your own supercharged deep conditioner.

After rinsing out the conditioner, apply your deep conditioner to your hair. You want a very liberal amount of deep conditioner to your hair, making sure all your hair from root to tip is covered. Work in portions or if you have your hair out, after application re-plait or re-twist. Cover with a plastic shower cap, and place a towel of fleecy material over and leave on for a minimum of 30 minutes. The towel or fleecy material provides a barrier against heat escaping for really deep penetration of nourishment. After your time is up, rinse out, without first opening your plaits or twists. Then style as usual.

It's not hair wash day, but you or your child are going swimming or playing a sport. What do you do to your hair and how do you make sure the water you're swimming in doesn't damage your hair? And the scalp sweating from non water based sport does not breed bacteria and make your hair smelly?

For swimming, dampen your hair with water from a spritz bottle, then apply some conditioner to all your hair however your hair is styled, a small handful, about 50 ml to 80 ml depending on the length of your hair. If your hair is not in any plaits or twists, please divide your hair into 5 big portions and plait up. This is highly important in avoiding tangled matted hair.

If you have extensions in, please only apply conditioner up to your own hair length. Then put a swim cap on if you can and go swimming. What the conditioner does is create a sort of barrier to help prevent the chlorine or salt or other molecules floating around in the pool from getting into your hair shaft, causing dryness which leads to breakage. Any water will open the hair cuticle.

We need to be sure we control what is entering our hair shaft. Wearing a swim cap, regardless of whether it fits properly or not, prevents the conditioner from being washed out almost instantly. Once swimming is done, apply some more conditioner and rinse through thoroughly, keeping your hair as it was when it went under the swim cap. Then apply a hair nourishing and moisturising cream to hair, paying special attention to the scalp. *Ommi's Beauty Nourishing Hair Cream* will work beautifully here.   If it's hair wash day then proceed to wash. If it is not, and hair needs styling, then proceed with usual hair styling.

If you are going to the gym or doing a non water based sport, then seal and nourish hair with oil that has essential oils in it. *Ommi's Beauty Liquid Gold Hair Oil* would be perfect for this job. Essential oils help prevent bacterial, fungal or viral growth taking place. Sweaty scalps are dark and damp, ideal growing grounds for microorganisms. Even if you are washing your hair afterwards it is still ideal to use the oil. Not only do essential oils help prevent growth of microorganisms, they help clean out our pores and hair follicles, they deliver essential nutrients to the scalp, hair bulb, hair root and hair shaft, and they boost your hair growth and hair health.

What better time to put oils in than when our pores and follicles are open and receptive due to exercise. For non-Afro hair, this is a brilliant way to use a lighter oil for pre-pooing whilst delivering amazing goodness to scalp and hair. *Ommi's Beauty Hairssential Hair Growth Oil* is a great oil to use for this purpose. I have used my experience and years as an aroma therapist and beauty therapist to put together a concentrated oil that packs a punch, for boosting hair growth whilst ridding scalp of bad microorganisms and preserving the Ph of the acid mantle of the scalp. Alternatively, you can buy one you prefer.

Do the above each time you are doing vigorous exercise, and if it's hair wash day, then, when done, proceed with hair wash day routine.

Washing your hair whilst it is plaited is not a recommendation that I would suggest, but if you have to, then you must, and here is some advice on how best to do that.

Wet your hair all over; apply conditioner to all your hair. If you have cornrows, leave it to sit for about 30 minutes. Then gently massage your scalp, working in between the plaits if you can. If not, try and move your whole scalp. Then thoroughly rinse out, and repeat if necessary.

Or you could use shampoo for a second wash if you feel your hair needs it, and then condition again after your shampoo wash. If you have single braids in, after you have applied the conditioner, work in portions and massage your scalp, making sure to not put too much pressure (scratching) on the base of your plaits. For each portion you are working on, make sure you hold all the plaits in that portion, lift the plaits towards your scalp, reducing the pressure on the scalp, and massage your scalp to get it clean.

Once you have done all your hair, rinse thoroughly. Repeat if necessary or use shampoo for second wash and then re-condition. After washing, apply your hair butter, cream, or oil to your scalp and work it into your hair plaits right up to where your own hair ends. If we don't nourish our hair in extensions the hair will become dry and brittle and have the 'crisp effect', as the extensions absorb moisture and the weather causes moisture to evaporate from our hair. We don't

98

want the 'crisp effect', as having extensions in is a protective hairstyle and supposed to help our hair to grow.

I tell you a short story about how healthy hair practices can make a vast difference to your hair length and how well it looks. My daughter, at 13 yrs, had hair that was waist length, about 30 inches long. It was then that she decided she did not want me to look after and style her hair. She wanted to do it herself. Suffice to say, her hair became a tangled mess, and in a space of six to eight months her hair went from being about 30 inches long to about 4 inches short, as it became so matted that I had to cut it all off and was ceremoniously taken off the mother of the year list.

For the next 18 months she refused to listen to any hair advice that I had to give, to my utter frustration. At my wits end I had an 'ah-ha' moment, and that was "Challenge her, compete with her." The first opportunity I had, I casually challenged her into a hair growth competition, flippantly stating that my hair would be twice as long as her hair in the next 6 months, with all my healthy hair practices. That was it! She secretly started carrying out all the hair advice I had been throwing at her the past months. Within 3 months her hair was the same length as mine, (she has an accelerated hair growth cycle), and within 6 it was twice the length of mine. Now her hair is about 25 inches long after 18 months of healthy hair practices.

I can now rest easy as a mom, knowing that she is taking good care of her hair.

Chapter 5

Hairstyles and How to Care for Them

Women and men wear their hair in all sorts of different, intriguing, amazing and beautiful hairstyles. In this chapter I'm going to give you details on how to care for your hair in the different hairstyles, give you information on what the different hairstyles are, and the knowledge of how to create a simple plait and a simple twist.

Why are hairstyles so important for hair? The importance comes from knowing how the different hairstyles affect our hair. Some are very beneficial to the long term health of our hair, while others may or may not be, depending on how they are done. We also have to bear in mind that the climate you live in will affect your hair. The best seasons for most hair types are autumn and spring if you are in Europe and at the beginning and end of the rainy season if you are in Africa.

These seasonal times are perfect for our hair because the air temperature is not too far off our body temperature and the moisture level in the atmosphere is just about enough. During winter the air temperature is too cold and freezes the moisture in our hair, making it prone to breaking. In the summer and at the height of the dry season, the temperature of the atmosphere is too high, causing our hair cuticles to open up, making the moisture in our hair evaporate, and thus causing dry brittle hair. So be aware of your climate change as this can have drastic effects on your hair. Take precautions on how to style and protect (if the weather warrants it) your hair whatever the season. The hairstyles below will help you do that.

So let's start with a couple of types of hairstyles that might need a bit more explaining.

Protective hairstyles: this is a group of hairstyles that protect your hair from stress and damage. The hairstyle mostly involves your hair, especially the ends, being plaited and or tucked/ folded away. It can be done in so many different ways, shapes and forms. This form of hairstyle protects mostly from the environmental heat and cold stress, that affects every race on this planet. Afro hair has the most surface area for moisture loss, so it benefits most from this type of hair styling. However, because hair is hair, and structurally all hair is the same, all hair will benefit greatly from this hairstyle, even men's hair. Heat stress evaporates moisture from your hair strands, making them dry and brittle. Cold stress freezes moisture in your hair strands, making them stiff and brittle. Protective hairstyling helps you to keep your hair strands close to your scalp, utilising the heat from your head, to keep your hair strands at optimum temperature to prevent breakage. This form of hairstyle is very good if you are trying to grow length. This applies to all hair types and all races.

Ever wondered why your Caucasian friend who always wears her hair in a bun is always saying her hair keeps growing like crazy, or why Black guys and ladies with dreads, who cover their hair all the time, or Asian men who wear turbans have really long hair, or Black ladies who wear correctly applied extensions have long hair? Here are some examples of protective hairstyles. Wearing head wraps are one of the best ways to protect your hair and braids and cornrows are the best protective hairstyles. Go onto the links below to learn how do a few of my favourite head wrap styles. As well as keeping your hair close to your scalp, they also prevent heat loss from your head, keeping more heat circulating around all of your hair.

I do love a good head wrap.

https://www.youtube.com/watch?v=ha6iX...

https://www.youtube.com/watch?v=Tw6xn...

Protective hairstyles should be worn according to your hair growth journey. If you are after increasing the length of your hair, then you must consider wearing them a lot of the time. If you want to maintain your hair health, then 3 to 7 days a month should suffice.

Low manipulation hairstyles: these are hairstyles that involve the bare minimum of moving your hair about. All protective hairstyling falls under low manipulation hairstyles as well. So when I say low manipulation/ bare minimum of movement of your hair, what do I mean? This is when you style your hair (whilst it is wet), then let it dry and then barely touch it or do not do anything to it for a period of time. Basically, less time hands or hair combs spend in your hair. So for me what does that look like? After I wash, condition and moisturise my hair, I set it how I would like it to look. That would look like either 3 or 4 cornrows on my head in the direction in which I'd like my hair to fall and if that was the curl pattern I wanted to sport for that week. Or it'll be single-plait-twists; normally about 6 to 10 plaits, again plaited in the general direction in which I'd like my hair to fall. I would then leave that on my hair for a minimum of 24hrs, but normally for about 2 to 3 days. If I'm not going out or meeting friends, then I would prolong the period of setting my hair. These styles used are protective hairstyles, and so the longer time hair is in these hairstyles the better it is for the hair.

Once I am ready to open my hair I would do so using only my fingers and being gentle with my hair as I undo it, trying to preserve the curl pattern created, and style it. Now, once it is styled I would not touch my hair until bedtime, and this will be to twist it into 3 or 5 big twists following my bedtime routine and using my fingers only. The fact that I didn't touch my hair throughout the day, didn't put any combs through it at any point, nor will I put any combs through it until hair wash day, is what I mean by low manipulation.

One can still use hair accessories like curbie grips, hair pins and hair clips to hold low manipulation hairstyles in place. The longer the period of time your hands and combs are away from your hair the better it is for your hair. These hairstyles also have the exact same benefits for hair of other races too. So feel free to try it out too, especially if you are not Black.

All plaited and braided extension hairstyles fall into this category. Dreadlocks/ Rasta hairstyles also fall into this category. As I go through the different hairstyles below I will show you how you can incorporate low manipulation into any hairstyle, and why is this beneficial for your hair. The greatest benefit it offers is little to no stress on your hair strands. And with little to no stress on your hair strands there is a very minimal chance of damage to your strands by manipulation. This lack of damage will help keep your hair healthy and retain length. If you want to grow your hair then you want to nourish your hair well, from the inside and outside, and then practise protective and low manipulation hairstyles. If you do this your hair length will surprise you.

Naturally Straight and Chemically processed hair

Permed/ Straightened, Keratin Blow-dried, Curled (wet or dry) and Texturised hair

Chemically Processed Hair

These hairstyles are achieved by using an alkaline based product, that enters the cortex of the hair shaft, to break down the disulfide bonds in the hair and reform them to the way we place the hair. All hair straightening and curling chemicals work on this principle. With a texturizer the product just weakens the bonds so the curls hang a bit looser. This is the process for all hair types for ALL races. With the curly perm you are placing the hair in curling rods so the disulfide bonds reform to the shape of the curling rod. However, with kinky curly Afro hair that you are straightening, you will be combing the hair straight so that the protein bonds reform straight. Same principle, different method. There are a lot of different products out there that help you achieve these results.

Go with what you know or what has been recommended by people you trust. Since we are using a chemical product that softens and opens up our hair cuticle, to work inside on a cellular level, stripping of nutrients, reduction of strength and moisture loss will occur. People with chemically processed hair need to be extra vigilant in trying to take care of their hair, as it dries out fast, easily making the hair more prone to breakage and split ends.

Chemically processed hair needs strengthening treatments and deep conditioning treatments.

Naturally Straight/Pressed/ Flat Ironed/ Hot Combed Hair

This hairstyle is achieved by using hot cast iron styling tongs and or combs and electric straighteners. The aim is to use heat to get the hair as straight as possible without permanently destroying the disulfide bonds in the hair shafts. This is more beneficial than chemical straightening. However, this means that once the hair is wet, and this includes humidity in the air, it will revert back to its normal curly state. (Which is why all women with this type of hairstyle worry about the weather, and if rain suddenly pours down they run for shelter as if a herd of wildebeests were chasing them, and any shelter will do. I was guilty of doing this too. I still am, even though I'm natural now.)

This is a good introduction to straight hair hairstyles for young children. Please, if you are unsure of proper technique, go to a professional to have it done, to avoid any burns. Your hair will remain straight until water or humidity makes it curly again; whichever happens first.

As this hairstyle is affected by water, you don't want to be using any moisture laden products. Preferably light oils to add shine, by sealing hair shafts and adding nourishment to scalp.

The constant application of heat to the hair, however, can be very drying, and the lack of moisture (water) application to the hair can eventually lead to dry brittle hair that breaks easily and has a lot of split ends. Extra care should be taken when washing and conditioning, a deep conditioner should always be used every wash day and hair should be washed once a week, maximum 10 day span. Anymore and your hair will become too dry, like a crisp.

Those with naturally straight hair that do not use heat to straighten their hair, just need to follow the nighttime and daytime routine below and the healthy hair practices in this book, adapting these practices to their specific hair type.

Your nighttime and daytime routine should look something like this:

Nighttime: First night after straightening, wrap hair and scarf before bed. Hair wrapping is a technique used to secure hair at night. Use a wide-toothed brush with protected tips. Start at the crown of your head and brush all your hair out into a bowl-like shape (the bottom of the bowl will be the crown of your head). Starting back at the crown of your head, brush your hair flat to your scalp, in a spiral, from crown to hair-line. Do this slowly to make sure you get all your hair to stay flat to your scalp, using your other hand to stop your hair from falling out of place. Second night will be time to add the light oil to your scalp, sparingly, and then massage it through whilst running your fingers to the ends of your hair.

I am assuming that you would be straightening your hair after washing, conditioning and adding suitable products to your hair and scalp to enhance hair and aid straightening. If you haven't then you may want to oil your scalp the first night. Then wrap your hair and scarf, and you are ready for bed. You want to add oil to scalp and hair on alternate days.

Daytime: brush out your wrapped hair and style in desired style. If you are using straighteners, try to always use them on the morning after the night you have applied oil to your hair, as this will help to protect your hair from the heat.

If after a few days your hair is starting to curl you can blow dry your hair or use some electric straighteners to redo the hair when it's not wash-day.

Black Natural - Curly or Kinky Hairstyle

What is Black natural hairstyle? It is the hairstyle where Black women and men wear their hair, as it grows out of the hair follicles, without any chemical processing. Key here is no chemical processing, so Black women who wear weaves, wigs, braids, or their hair is in dreadlocks still have natural hair in their braids and dreadlocks, and underneath the weaves and wigs, as long as there is no chemical processing of the hair that grows out of their hair follicles. How to care for this hair has baffled Black people as well as every other race alike for centuries. I will not say the learning is over, because I don't think we ever stop learning and if you do, you end up with a very closed mindset, not expanding or growing at all. But I can shed some light and help you along your way to 'good hair', as we are ever growing, evolving and changing.

If you want your natural hair to look healthy, whatever your hair length, this is where you need to sit up and take notes. Can I just say, if you have trashed your hair over time or merely just not taken good care of your hair, doing the exercises in here isn't going to create an instant miracle. 'Good hair' is achieved, over time, with consistent practice. It takes about 28 to 30 days for the effects of any new practice to be seen in your hair. So invest a few minutes every day in your hair and the results will speak for themselves.

So what should your natural hair care routine look like?

Realistically you should be washing your hair every 7 to 10 days. Waiting longer than 10 days leaves your hair open to dryness and a buildup of dead skin cells. You should never style your hair unless it is wet from washing or from spritzing it with water for a mid-current-style change. Always remember the piece of crisp and slice of potato analogy and which one is easier to manipulate without breaking. Aim for your hair to always be the slice of potato when you are combing or styling your hair. Style as you wish using products that benefit your hair and scalp.

At nighttime you want be placing your hair in a protective style, twists or plaits, if it's not already in one, and a satin or silk scarf or bonnet over your hair to stop friction and moisture absorption by bed sheets, before sleeping.

Nighttime and daytime routines naturally straight or chemically straightened hair

What should your nighttime routine look like? You should always be aiming to protect your hair whilst you sleep. Protecting your hair from moisture loss and breakage is a must, and this goes for children as well. Our cotton bed sheets absorb nearly all moisture and oils from the hair, drying it out overnight. Ever wondered why your hair feels like straw when you miss out your scarfing? Or moms of curly haired children, you ever wondered why your children's hair feels dry and straw-like and is very matted every morning? Or ladies, you who don't scarf your hair, ever wondered why your hair takes up so much product every time? The best way to prevent this from happening is to use satin or silk pillowcases or to use a satin bonnet or silk scarf to cover your hair at night. The downside of using a satin or silk pillowcase is that your hair strands are not kept close to your scalp, keeping in the heat, protecting them from breakage as well by doing away with all friction. The satin bonnet or silk scarf works best for this purpose.   It keeps your hair close to your scalp, utilising your body's temperature to keep your hair supple, as well as preventing breakage and drying out.

For people who are not used to wearing something on their head at night, this will take some getting used to, but the benefits are well worth the perseverance. For young children, the earlier you start getting them used to having a sleeping scarf or bonnet on, the better.   For most Black people, wearing something on your hair at night is something that happens from infant stage, so it becomes part of daily life. Before you cover your hair, if it's long you should always fold your hair or wrap your hair.

Wrapping will be for people with naturally straight or chemically processed straight hair or hair that is straightened by flat iron, hot comb or straighteners. This will keep hair in a better shape for less hassle in the morning time, and it will actually help your hairstyle sit better. However, before you wrap or fold your hair at night you should always aim to moisturise and seal your hair.

By moisturise I mean adding some form of water and or leave-in conditioner (preferable both), so this is not for those who have flat ironed or hot combed their hair. I make my own leave-in conditioner that makes my hair touchably soft and keeps it well moisturised. The recipe is in the products chapter. I then seal my hair with a Hair Oil. You should keep it in the fridge as this helps prevent bacterial growth. The essential oils also help prevent bacterial growth, and the cooled temperature of your leave-in conditioner helps cool and refresh your scalp. You do not need to soak your hair. Work in portions and just mist your hair. Working in portions makes sure you treat all your hair to a moisture top up. Then you go in with your nourishing cream, then sealing oil. Hair types that need sealing are all Black hair types, and very thick or very curly non Black-hair. All other hair types are ok with just the leave-in conditioner. Use sealing oil that best suits your hair type, one that will be easily absorbed by your hair so it doesn't weigh it down. If your hair has a high porosity then this should be done every night or at least every other night. For low porosity or well sealed hair, this can be done 2 to 3 times a week. Then fold or wrap your hair and cover. Now your hair is all ready for bed.

Daytime routine

With the above nightly routine you really would not have to do much in the morning (low manipulation). If you have folded your hair, you would unfold and style your hair as usual.

If you have folded into small twists, cornrows or bantu-knots to create a curl pattern, then you'll undo those and use your fingers to style your hair, making sure to preserve your curls you have so lovingly created. If you have wrapped your hair, then brush it out, with a wide-toothed brush or comb, with protected tips, and style as usual. Or you can blow dry or straighten your hair if you so wish, but please do so without washing your hair. And voila... you are ready to start your day. Well, your hair is anyways.

Another good thing to add into your routine is a scalp massage. This is beneficial to your scalp and hair because it increases blood and lymph flow to and from your scalp. Increased blood flow means more oxygen and nutrients to your scalp and hair, fortifying and strengthening it, there by aiding better utilisation of the good-for-your-hair products. Increase lymph flow means more white blood cells in the area to fight off and take away any microorganisms and pathogens. This all helps to produce healthy hair and scalp. A 5-minute scalp massage a day is best. If you can do longer great. Ten minutes is ample, but for best results, 5 minutes minimum. Whatever time of day you do your scalp massage is up to you. It can also help with headache and migraine relief. Regular scalp massages with stimulating products are known to also help with stimulating <u>dormant</u> hair follicles. *Ommi's Beauty Hairssential Oil* will work brilliantly here.

Weaves, Crochet Braids, Wigs and Cornrows

Weaves or sew-ins and cornrow hairstyles are achieved by plaiting your natural hair close to your scalp. Now this can be done with or without extensions, which are synthetic strands of hair that are added to each individual cornrow or braid.

I remember getting my first weave done after my daughter was born. As the hairdresser was plaiting my hair before attaching the weave, I remembered asking her not to plait it so tight. She dismissively answered "If you don't want the weave to fall out I have to plait it tight! It has to be tight for it to last you." I remembered accepting her answer and dreading the situation it was putting me in, thinking "For the next week or so I'm going to have a constant headache, with a 3 month old baby!" At that time I didn't know better and this situation was "normal", as everyone I knew that had a weave, braids or cornrows went through the same thing. I was always made to feel I was the problem because I have a sensitive scalp. I accepted it, until I learned better.

My scalp being sensitive, and everyone around me, apart from my mother, blaming me for my sensitive scalp, saying my hair was too difficult to deal with, is what pushed me into the hairdressing field. It constantly irritated me, and I was determined to find a better way so I would not suffer the pain this misconception brought about. I also wanted to prove that you could have amazing weaves, braids and cornrows that last a long time, without the plaits being tight on your scalp. For that reason I learned to plait hair early, so I could do my own hair. The first time I plaited my own hair and went to school...., suffice to say that the plaits weren't all that good. I got teased immeasurably. This only made me more determined to find a better way.

For weave hairstyles, once the cornrows are done, then wefts of hair, normally made with human hair or synthetic hair, are sewn on top of the cornrows in a style that the client has asked for. This can be done on the whole head or just a few strips of hair wefts can be sewn in to give length and volume.

When it's just a few wefts sewn in, you want to moisturise the tracks/plaits with your leave-in conditioner at least every 2 to 3 days, depending on the dryness of your hair, and then seal with an oil that's suitable for your hair. When sealing make sure you place the oil along the full length of the track, above and below it. This is very important, as having these tracks put in does dry out the natural hair regardless of race. Sometimes the synthetic hair that is put into the tracks itches the scalp and may cause irritation (redness and flaking), the moisturisation and sealing helps prevent the itching and scalp irritation.

Your nighttime and daytime routine should be as above. And when it comes to washing your hair please refer to the section on washing your hair while it's in braids.

If your hairstyle is a full head of weave, you will want to moisturise and seal at least once a week. This is because with all the extensions on top of your plaited hair, it doesn't give much room for your hair to dry quickly or breathe freely. You don't want your hair and scalp constantly moist as this will be ideal breeding ground for microorganisms. You want to use heavier oils with a few drops of essential oils in it, to maximise hair and scalp health. *Ommi's Beauty Nourishing Hair Cream or Ommi's Beauty Sealing Hair Butter* will work brilliantly here.

Please follow the nighttime and daytime routine in the above section for naturally straight or curly and chemically straightened hair. But instead of using your precious ingredients on your weave, which is hair that will be thrown away after, and honestly you don't need much to make a weave look good, you should get a hair serum from the shops, apply in portions, fold or wrap hair and then cover before bed. Use your good-for-your-hair products on your scalp only.

When it is time to wash your hair, please follow the guidelines for washing your hair whilst it is plaited. After you have washed your hair, please apply your butters and or oils to your scalp, in-between the tracks of your weave. Make sure you cover your entire scalp. Apply a small amount of olive oil (about a 50 pence size) to your hands and work it all throughout the hair. This is all the oil you need for your weave. Then apply some hair serum and blow dry or set with rollers and sit under the drier. This care is for human hair weaves. If you have a synthetic hair weave, you pretty much won't be able to do anything with it or even wash it without ruining it. All you need to do is apply a small amount of hair serum to the hair every 2 to 3 days. So just leave it be and focus on your scalp care, of moisturising and sealing once weekly.

For wig styling, most Black people would normally plait their hair in cornrows and put the wig upon it daily. It is ideal if you are going to be wearing a wig constantly that you plait your hair underneath. This helps to protect your natural hair, as you would have the cornrows in for a period of time. So essentially, your hair care routine would be to follow the one for plaited hair below.

However, you can use some of the tips above for weaves to care for your wig, or you can care for and style it as you wish. Do make sure that your wig fits your head perfectly, as in imperfect fit will lead to the wig moving about, causing friction to your natural hair. This friction will produce breakage to your hair. Also, always try and wear a satin wig cap under your wig regardless of fit to reduce moisture absorption and friction.

For cornrows, once your hair is plaited you need to make sure it's not too tight, as this will hamper any care for the hair that is needed. The care advice below will be for any style of cornrows, regardless of whether your plaits are all your own hair or whether you have extensions plaited into your cornrows. When people have cornrows plaited they normally keep them in for anything from one to eight weeks and sometimes more.

Your cornrows should be washed about once every two to three weeks whilst plaited. Make sure you wash it in the morning so that it has the whole day to dry, or sit under the dryer. If you have a dry scalp condition (or very bad dandruff) you will need to wash your hair every one to two weeks and you will need to wash your hair with the plaits OUT preferably. This will ensure that all that dead dry skin is able to slide off the hair shafts instead of getting trapped in the plaited hair.

Your nighttime care will be to use a hair oil in-between all the rows every night before bed. This helps keep your scalp moisturised, nourish your hair follicles, strengthen your hair shaft and help prevent build-up and breakage. Then you need to scarf your hair at night to keep your hair neat and prevent the oils from being absorbed by your cotton bed sheets. Then in the morning, once a week, you will spray your hair with your leave-in conditioner so that your hair is a little damp, and apply some form of nourishing hair cream to your scalp (in between the rows) and a sealing butter over the hair to seal the moisture in. Endeavour to do this in the morning so that your hair has all day to dry, as plaited hair tends to hold on to moisture much longer, and therefore takes longer to dry.

When it is time to take your cornrows out, make sure you use some hair oil in between the rows, a fair amount, this is to give slippage, to minimise the damage caused by the manipulation of undoing the cornrows. After applying a generous amount of oil, you then want to wet your hair with water, just plain water, until your hair is just damp, NOT dripping wet, and then proceed with taking the cornrows out. Once out and ready to wash, follow the hair wash routine in 'hair wash day'. Always wash your hair in between cornrow styles.

Washing and conditioning adds moisture which helps keep hair supple and aids manoeuvrability, preventing breakage. It's not advisable to plait cornrows again straight after taking one lot out, as hair will be very dry and tangled. It will hurt the scalp more, as hair will be full of knots and the dryness will make the knots hard to be detangled, causing a lot of breakage.

However, if you follow the above hair care routine and use good-for-your-hair products, you may just about be able to get away with redoing your cornrows straight after taking one set out. If you do this make sure it's only one or two weeks in-between plaiting to avoid smelly hair. You should also be mindful of the amount of fluff at the base of each cornrow.

Here is a short how-to on cornrows and single plaits, so that you can try out doing a basic cornrow and a basic single plait. Cornrows are a popular West African style of braiding the hair along the scalp. The name was derived from the fact that, a cornrow braid well done, looks like two rows of corn on a cob. The corn kernels grow in the same neat symmetrical way as the braid on the head. As young girls living in West Africa you are taught how to braid hair from the moment you have your first doll. It is frowned upon if a young girl does not know how to plait her own hair and that of her little sisters by the age of 12. Cornrows are also known as "underhand track braids". It's a traditional art and anyone who has the patience can learn it, but it takes some time and skill to master.

This lesson will help you get started with the basics whilst avoiding some beginner's mistakes.

Cornrow Plaiting

1. Section off part of the hair that you want to plait, in the direction you want the cornrow to follow. The rest of the hair that is not part of the plait, tie it away, moving all other hair out of the way.

2. At where you want the cornrow to start, grab a small cross-section of the hair and divide into 3 equal strands/parts. Take only a little bit and don't pull too hard on the hair.

3. Hold the 3 equal strands separate and weave them around each other alternatively once.

4. Holding the far left strand separate from the other two, reach down with your left hand and grab a small amount of hair from the area to be cornrowed. Merge this new hair completely with the left strand so it becomes one.

5. Now weave it under the middle strand and over the right strand.

6. Holding the far right strand separate from the other 2, reach down with your right hand and grab a small amount of hair from the area to be cornrowed. Merge this new hair completely with the right strand so it becomes one.

7. Now weave it under the middle strand and over the left strand.

8. Continue this alternate grabbing of hair from the area being cornrowed until no hair from the scalp is left out. As you are adding the hair try not to pull the hair tightly at the root.

9. Plait the end of the hair by continuing the alternative left strand under the middle and over the right strand, then right strand under the middle and over the left strand until you have no more hair to plait.

10. For hair that may come undone quickly, secure with an elastic band made specifically for hair, a scrunchie or a hair clip.

Single Plaits Plaiting

1. Section off the portion of hair that you would like to plait into a single plait.

2. Separate that portion into 3 equal strands/parts.

3. Weave the left strand under the middle and over the right strand.

4. Then weave the right strand under the middle and over the left strand.

5. Continue this alternative weaving until you have no more hair to plait.

6. For hair that may come undone quickly, secure with an elastic band specifically for hair, a scrunchie or a hair clip.

Single Braids and Dreadlocks

Braided hairstyles are achieved by portioning your hair. These can be from large (one big braid) to very very small (micro braids). The braid is achieved by dividing the portion into 3 parts and weaving them in and out of each other to create a braid. The braid can be made using just your own hair or adding in extension hair to the portion to add length and volume.

When people have braids done, they are planning on keeping it in for a minimum of about 8 weeks to as long as 12 to 16 weeks. The reason for this lengthy time in the hair is because, when people do single braids, they more often than not do them quite small. This is for a number of reasons, the one main reason being so that the braided style simulates your natural hair being tangle free and easy to style.

To achieve these styles is often a costly and lengthy process. It can cost anything from £50 up to and more than £250. Celebrities will pay much more than this, and a style can take anything from 2 to 8hrs plus to complete. I have even done hairstyles that have taken 2 days to complete. After one has spent all that time in a hairdresser's chair and spent all that money, there is no desire to go through that process again anytime soon, so you can understand why people keep their braids in for that long.

This section is all about helping you care for your braids, to make sure it doesn't have a negative effect on your natural hair. More often than not, people who have braids often or all the time tend to suffer from traction-alopecia either during the period that they are wearing braids or in later years. One of the major causes of traction-alopecia in braided hair is plaits that are too tight. The second major reason is the weight of the extension hair being added to the portion of natural hair. The advice in this section will aim to help you prevent hair loss and keep your hair growing and staying healthy.

The first tip will be to use lighter in weight hair extensions and not put too much extension hair in each portion. Make sure your hair portion can support the hair extensions being put in. Second tip will be to make sure the hairdresser does not plait the hair portions too tight. Most of the time the braids are started off quite tight, but it doesn't seem to hurt or affect your scalp until near the end. This is because the braids are being plaited tighter than the movement of your scalp.

It's not until near the end of plaiting when your scalp has no movement whatsoever left that we feel the pain. To avoid this tightness and pain, the 1st half of the hair needs to be plaited close to the scalp but still loose enough to allow movement of the scalp. Then the last half of the hair can be braided more tightly based on what you or the client can bear and the movement left in the scalp. There is this misconception amongst the Black community that if your hair is not as tight as it can possibly be then your hair is not neat or beautiful. We can have neat and beautiful hair without it being tight.

Once your braids are in, you will want to moisturise your scalp about twice a week, or at the very least once a week with a nourishing cream. This is best done at night time, before tying your hair up for bed. You should also include a head massage for about 5 to 10 minutes long. This helps stimulate the blood and lymph flow to the scalp, encouraging growth. Then about twice a week, always in the morning, you want to spritz your hair until damp with water, then use a small amount of a nourishing cream and go over each individual plait up to where your own hair ends. Even though your hair is all plaited up it still needs care. You should work the cream into to each plait right up to where your hair tip is.

If you have small to really small plaits, do this in portions of plaits grouped together in manageable sizes that will allow you to make sure each plait is damp and has some nourishing cream through it, thus ensuring that your own hair in each plait is being taken care of.

Tip: you don't need to dampen and nourish the extension bit that does not have your natural hair in it. The extension bit that goes past your natural hair... no need to worry about that.

If you do this for the length of time you have your braids in, you will find you have less knots and tangles when you undo your braids, and your hair will be in a much better condition.

One of the reasons braids are so popular is, once done it's a protective, low manipulation, and low maintenance hairstyle that helps your hair to grow. The reason your hair grows is because of the prior two reasons. However, once the braids are out the hair is more often than not very dry, due to the extensions drawing out all the moisture from your hair. Even if you don't have extensions in, and your braids are all your natural hair, and you don't moisturise and nourish your braids, your hair will still end up being very dry, as hair will naturally lose moisture over time, and unless it is replenished manually your hair will remain dry.

The dreadlock hairstyle is a long standing hairstyle, but only really burst into mainstream in the 1970s when Bob Marley and the Wailers become famous. Dreads are steeped in history. The first recorded archeological proof came when mummies from Egypt were dug up with their dreads still intact. Some believe they might have originated in India and that India is the spiritual home of dreads. Dreads have been worn for many centuries and by many cultures, but it was not until the last 10 years that dreadlocks became a style with neater smaller locks, and women started to wear the style more.

Some women have them in very small strand-like styles. It was not until dreads were worn in sizes smaller and neater that the prejudice of dreads being just unkempt hair started to drop. I remember as a kid, seeing Rastafarians and thinking "their hair looks really unkempt." That was because I didn't know any better and I didn't really know these individuals. Today dreads are done in salons across the world, and are a hairstyle that is ingrained in the Beauty industry now. With more women wearing them, the need to actually still have luscious hair even if they are in dreads is apparent.

In this section I help you to maintain the lusciousness of your dreads.

As we have established in this book, good scalp care and moisture levels in our hair strands, no matter your hairstyle, is key in maintaining and growing 'good hair'. One of the biggest help to dreads will be moisture. Dreads is a hairstyle that can be drier than most. This is because all the naturally shed hair is 'locked' in with the growing hair, and over time that shed hair cuticles do not close, so loses moisture quickly and easily and this is what give dreads that rough straw-like feel and look. So for people with dread hairstyles, your spritz bottle with just water should be your best friend.

Dread leave-in Conditioner mix. In a 250 ml spritz bottle add: 1 tsb of Jojoba oil; 3 drops of Lavender; 3 drops of Peppermint. Fill with water. Shake vigorously and spray hair. Always shake vigorously before using.

Each week you want to be moisturising your scalp with a nourishing cream at least 3 times. You should use the cream all over your scalp, and give yourself a scalp massage for about 5 minutes. The massage increases blood flow to the area, keeping your scalp in tip top condition, and aids in absorbing the nutrients in the nourishing cream.

Daytime routine: spritz your hair with your water and oil leave-in conditioner until each strand is damp. Apply a small amount of hair oil to all strands of your hair from root to tip. *Ommi's Beauty Liquid Gold Hair Oil* would work perfectly here. This can be done without precision, just making sure that all your hair is covered. This should be done at least every other day, and doing it in the morning makes sure your hair is moisturised all day. On the in between days just get up and go. Now, that's something all of us would like.

Nighttime routine; apply a nourishing cream to scalp and drag the cream down your dread strands. Don't worry too much about applying cream to the last 3rd of your strands, and if you are doing the above daytime routine that portion of your hair will be moisturized anyways. (Dreadlocks strands don't suffer from breakage due to the fact that all the shed hair and growing hair are 'locked' together making it a thick continuous strand that is hard to break, compared to one normal strand of hair.) Then give yourself a scalp massage. Afterwards, put your hair up, wrap it around your head and scarf your hair or simply put your satin bonnet on and go to bed.

When you do your nighttime routine, you don't need to do your daytime routine. My advice would be to alternate your days, so your week would look something like this; Monday, night time routine, Wednesday, daytime routine, Friday, night time routine, Sunday, daytime routine. This way your hair is always moisturized and looking luscious.

When it's time to wash your hair you would need to follow the hair wash routine for plaited hair in the hair wash chapter.

Twists and Bantu Knots, colloquially known as 'Chicken Poo Poo'

Twists and Bantu Knots are hairstyles that are used to set hair for other curly hairstyles. They involve taking a portion of hair and twisting it round and round until it makes a coil - bantu knots; or taking a portion of your hair, dividing it into 2 or 3 smaller portions and twisting those round each other to create a twist. Bantu knots are known as 'chicken poo poo' in

Liberia because of the way it coils and the way it sits on your head, slightly resembling a chicken's poo on the ground. You leave them in for a minimum of 8 to 24hrs, so overnight or a full day. Then you undo them and style your hair with the curls they have created. This can be done on any hair type, straight, wavy, curly or kinky hair. It can help you get a more defined curl pattern.

Most Black women who have natural hair will use some form of this hair styling to set their curls. Which one you use depends entirely on personal preference of how you want your curls to look and sit. I tend to use the twists more for my hair styling. This hair styling can be done on other hairstyles, to change up or enhance them. For example, you can twist or put into bantu knots, braided hair, dreadlocks, weaves and wigs.

As this hairstyle is an enhancement hairstyle, you would care for your hair with the haircare routine of your foundation style and hair type.

Threaded Hairstyle

This is a typically West African hairstyle, however different forms of it are practiced all over Africa. This style is created using thread made of cotton, linen, or plastic. The hair is portioned into whatever size portions the wearer would like. Each portion of hair is then wrapped with thread from the root, with barely any gaps in between each wrap, until the tip is reached, and a knot is tied at the end to secure it. Once each portion on the whole head is wrapped in thread, the portions are then twisted together to form a hairstyle.

This hair style would normally be worn for about 2 to 4 weeks. Now, this form of hair styling is being used as a way to straighten curly to kinky hair without any heat. This can be done in large or small portions, and once hair is dry the thread is then removed to reveal the dry straightened hair, to style as one chooses.

This will be used as a hair styling tool just like twists and bantu knots.

MEN'S - Natural, Long, Cut & Shaped or Texturized

Men's scalp and hair need the same care and nutrition that ladies' do, because the cellular structure and function of the scalp and hair is not any different from women's. Please follow the hair care routine for any of the previous hairstyles if that is the hair style you wear. Black men who have medium to long natural hair and are trying to retain length, you would need to follow the hair care routine for Black Natural Curly or Kinky hair or that for braided or cornrow styles, or that of chemically processed hair if your hair is processed and long or short.

For cut texturised hair, which is chemically processed hair as well, your hair care will be slightly different.

Nighttime: wash hair, then use good hair oil or hair cream on hair and scalp, and massage scalp for at least 5 minutes, but 10 minutes is even better. Brush into style, tie hair with Do-rag and sleep.

Day time: remove Do-rag when ready and it's all done. For men who keep their hair natural and low to medium-ish length; if you wash your hair everyday then you may want to oil or cream your hair and scalp in the morning after you wash it, then style. Nighttime would be a good time to do your scalp massage for optimum scalp and hair health.

Please treat your hair and scalp to a proper treatment at least once a month. You can choose any from the treatment section. It is good to have and follow a good hair care routine to keep your scalp and hair in optimum condition.

Chapter 6

Conclusion

What is good hair?
More importantly, "What is your perception of good hair?"

I have come to realise that the statement of 'good hair' is just a myth, as everyone has good hair on their head, regardless of race, colour or origin. Everyone has 'good hair' growing out of their scalp, on their head. That elusive statement of 'good hair' is in reality, 'good looking hair', which is the manifestation of healthy hair practices. With that reality, it then makes it possible for anyone with hair from any race, colour or origin to achieve 'good looking hair'. Your curl pattern or the straightness of your hair is not what gives you 'good hair', nor do these have any impact on how healthy your hair is. It is what you do to your hair and how you treat it that makes it healthy or not healthy.

Our perception of 'good hair' is what determines how we feel about our hair. That perception is shaped solely by external factors. How we treat that hair and how well we take care of it, is a whole different matter.

At the end of the day, there is just healthy hair, and unhealthy hair. All manner of unhealthy practices will produce unhealthy hair, in just the same way as all manner of healthy practices will produce healthy hair. What we want to strive for, at all times, is to have healthy hair, regardless of age, race, colour or origin.

Always use good-for-your-hair-products on your hair. Investing some money and a little bit of time each day in your hair will invariably produce healthy results. If you feel a product is not working for your hair, stop using it immediately; give it to someone else who might have better results, or just throw it away.

Be good to your hair and it will be good to you, regardless of your race, colour, or origin. In today's society our differences are used to separate us rather than celebrate our uniqueness. By celebrating our uniqueness and realising our similarities we are able to embrace the world and strive for a united cause, prosperity, survival and a healthy planet. I hope I have managed to show you that there is so much more similarity in us then there is difference. We need to embrace the similarities, accept the differences, celebrate the oneness in life, serve others and the world, and put our best self forward with healthy good looking hair and scalp.

#HairIsHair #HIH #YourBestBeautiful

Email ommisbeauty2007@gmail.com with the discount code HAIRISHAIR to get 20% off your first order for products.

Click this link to buy your Arbonne products http://www.EugeniaShaw.arbonne.com

To get 20% for all Arbonne products for a year email ommisbeauty2007@gmail.com and place in the subject area ARBONNE DISCOUNT.

For the specialist products in the recipes in this book you can purchase them at Akoma. Here is a link to their website https://www.akomaskincare.co.uk. Use the discount code HAIRISHAIR and get 15% off on your first order.

Come be a part of our hair community on Facebook, search 'Hair is Hair' Healthy Hair Masterclass. Look forward to connecting with you on there.

Thank you so very much for taking the time to read my book. I sincerely hope it has given you some insight and guidance on how to manage your hair, for your hair to be its Best Beautiful version always.

For me to improve the next version of this book and any future books I write, I would appreciate your feedback.

A helpful review on Amazon, sharing your thoughts about the book, would be amazing.

Thank you and have a blessed day xx
Eugenia Shaw

Bibliography

These are few of the references that contributed to my knowledge when I was writing this book. Over my years in the Beauty Industry and during my training years I have done extensive research using books and online sources, never really thinking I'd be writing about my knowledge one day. My personal experience and research knowledge gave me the base to draw on for this book. I will never stop learning and look forward to learn something new every day. Knowledge opens the mind and expands awareness.

Lorraine Nordmann and Marian Newman, *The Foundation, Beauty Therapy, all editions.*

Julia Lawless, *The Encyclopedia of Essential Oils, all editions.*

The Trichological Society, www.hairscientists.org

Printed in Great Britain
by Amazon